"The sound, solid advice and information in this book is a refreshing change to all the 'quick fixes' out there. *Thin in 10* actually gives you a plan that works. It's all broken down into 10 minute (or less) bite-size steps that anyone can get results from!"
—*Michele Olson, PhD, professor of exercise science at Auburn University—Montgomery*

"An easy-to-read guide to weight loss, and though there is plenty of research to back up the *Thin in 10* method, you won't get lost in science or stats; instead you'll get a road map to results."
—*Dr. Karen Koffler, medical director of Canyon Ranch in Miami Beach, FL*

"The exercises in this book are safe, effective, and offer great progressions for all levels—whether you are just starting out or have been working out for years . . . a full range of options for everyone."
—*Amy Dixon, exercise physiologist, Los Angeles celebrity trainer and creator of numerous best-selling fitness DVDs.*

"Thank you for not telling readers to give up carbs or other foods groups or, more importantly, food they love. Finally, a diet plan that is sensible and makes sense! Even as a super busy mom with my own business and two kids I could cook all of the recipes and feed my entire family with them—no complaints!"
—*Tracey Mallet, international fitness presenter and creator of the Booty Barre Method*

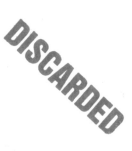

The
THIN IN
10

Weight-Loss
Plan

Transform Your Body (and Life!) in Minutes a Day

Jessica Smith *and*
Liz Neporent

SUNRISE
River Press

SUNRISE
River Press

Sunrise River Press
39966 Grand Avenue
North Branch, MN 55056
Phone: 651-277-1400 or 800-895-4585
Fax: 651-277-1203
www.sunriseriverpress.com

Edit by Corrine Casanova
Layout by Connie DeFlorin

ISBN 978-1-934716-35-9
Item No. SRP635

Library of Congress Cataloging-in-Publication Data

Smith, Jessica.
  Thin in 10 : the 10-minute weight-loss plan / by Jessica Smith & Liz Neporent.
     p. cm.
  Includes index.
  ISBN 978-1-934716-35-9
1. Weight loss--Popular works. 2. Exercise--Popular works. 3. Nutrition--Popular works. 4. Self-care, Health--Popular works. I. Neporent, Liz. II. Title. III. Title: Thin in ten.
  RM222.2.S62238 2012
  613.2'5--dc23

Printed in China
10 9 8 7 6 5 4 3 2 1

To my daughter, Skylar, the best piece of workout equipment ever
— Liz

To my husband, Guillermo, thank you for your love, support, and encouragement. And to my mom and dad, thanks for saving my very first "published" book ever—think I've come a long way from the story about the little girl who hated "Peas and Other Vegetables."
— Jessica

Acknowledgments

We had a lot of fun writing this book. That's thanks in large part to our wonderful agent, Linda Konner. She stuck with this project and found it the best possible home with Sunrise River Press and our terrific editor Karen Chernyaev. Thanks to you too, Karen, for your thoughtful and thorough edits.

To Tamilee Webb, one of the pioneers of the fitness industry, we offer our humble gratitude. We appreciate not only that you agreed to write our foreword but also your amazing contributions to the health and fitness world. Your sane, sensible—yet no-nonsense—approach to working out is something we strive to emulate.

We wish to thank all our clients, especially our *Thin In 10* focus group members. You helped us push and pull this program, and we know this book is better for your honest and insightful feedback. Readers will surely benefit from all your hard work. We also wish to acknowledge the scientists whose research we've referenced throughout this book. We wanted our plan to be as evidence based as possible and, although science is constantly evolving, we've done our best to base our recommendations on the most current thinking available.

Of course, we'd be remiss if we didn't give a shout out to our respective friends and family. Liz wishes to thank Jessica for being such a fabulous coauthor and friend. Liz also feels lucky to have the greatest husband and daughter in the world, who support everything she does without complaint. And Jessica is honored to be working with her amazingly talented and prolific coauthor and dear friend, Liz, and the extremely multi-talented fitness PR guru Melissa McNeese.

Finally, thanks to you dear reader. We understand how much commitment it takes to lose weight, to get in shape, and to better your life. We hope you get everything you need to do just that. Please let us know how you're doing! Visit us at www.thinin10.com. You can check in, ask questions, and find info, tips, videos, and more that will help you achieve your goals.

Contents

Foreword

BY TAMILEE WEBB
STAR OF *BUNS OF STEEL* AND IDEA INSTRUCTOR OF THE YEAR

Lack of time is the number one excuse I hear from people about why they're not exercising. In this busy, overscheduled, multitasking world we live in, they simply don't have enough time to squeeze in a workout. I get that. Even though fitness is the way I make my living and exercise is obviously a priority for me, sometimes even I struggle to find a way to fit in my workouts.

That's why the information in this book is such a revelation. It's a sane, sensible program that shows you how to tackle losing weight 10 minutes at a time. Each workout is designed to supercharge your weight loss and shape-up potential in just 10 short minutes. It's a quick and efficient workout approach—plus there aren't any hidden time wasters like setting up equipment or getting to the gym.

I have always believed that anything you do to lose weight should have solid evidence to back it up; this ensures that you devote your precious time only to strategies that actually help you reach your goals. I'm happy to report that the *Thin in 10* style of working out meets my standards. As the pages that follow explain, there is plenty of research proving that short, intense workouts can be just as effective for burning fat and calories as long, slow workouts. And, as studies show, shorter, harder workouts may actually bestow a unique caloric advantage by revving up your metabolism so you continue to burn calories at a higher rate long after you've hit the showers. Plus, it's a lot easier to stick with since a 10-minute workout commitment is pretty much excuse proof!

As for the *Thin in 10* eating plan, I'm a fan of any diet—like this one— that promotes a good balance of nutrition and doesn't go overboard in limiting your calories or food choices. The bonus is that all of the recipes can be prepared in 10 minutes or less. Like a workout, a diet should be realistic and manageable over the long haul. This plan more than qualifies on those terms. (By the way, my favorite recipe is Pizza in a Flash, found in chapter 11. What's not to like about this healthy version of a fast-food indulgence?)

One unique aspect of the *Thin in 10* program is that it addresses all the other lifestyle factors that can affect weight loss. We are just finding out, for instance, how important adequate sleep seems to be for preventing a pileup of pounds; *Thin in 10* includes a detailed discussion of this idea and gives some fantastic advice on how to get a good night's sleep. Engineering movement into your day to burn calories beyond what you do in your workouts is also turning out to be a key component in successful weight loss. This book devotes a whole chapter to listing simple yet creative ways to build activity into your day. There's even an entire chapter's worth of advice on how to stay motivated so you stick with the program even during those inevitable periods when your resolve is weak.

This plan seems to account for everything you need to lose the weight and keep it off for good. As an expert in the field of health and fitness, I can tell you I give a lot of the same advice contained in this book to my clients and certainly follow many of the same principles it outlines in my own life. I think the premise of achieving the body of your dreams in 10-minute increments is realistic, especially if you follow a plan as focused as this one. So let go of any assumptions that successful weight loss means starving yourself or spending hours at the gym. Just give it 10 minutes and let the information in this book guide you to success.

Introduction

You may wonder how a 10-minutes-at-a-time approach to health and fitness can possibly help you lose weight and get in shape for good. You are probably thinking (like a lot of our focus group did at first) that 10 minutes doesn't sound like enough time to get anything of significance done, let alone achieve your weight-loss goals. But 10 minutes is the perfect chunk of time. For starters, it's easy for your brain to accept that you can handle 10 minutes of whatever it is you have to do. Also, plenty of evidence backs up the idea that 10 minutes of exercise at a time is more than enough to achieve some success. (More about that in just a bit.) Finally, we know it works, because, as creators of the *Thin in 10* program, we have both experienced the success for ourselves.

Jessica and Liz Get Personal

Both of us are successful fitness professionals. Jessica is a certified personal trainer and one of the best-known fitness instructors in the country. She's the star of best-selling exercise videos that have sold more than 7 million copies to date. She's even appeared on over 40 million Kellogg's cereal boxes as the fitness expert for "10-Minute Solution," a popular series of exercise DVDs. Liz is also a certified personal trainer and holds a master's degree in exercise physiology. She's an emeritus board member, faculty member, and spokesperson for the American Council on Exercise, one of the most influential fitness consumer groups in the world. We are both lifelong exercisers, eat well, and in general, practice what we preach.

From the sound of it, you'd think the two of us are so into fitness we must have been born with perfect bodies and never once worried about weight. Wrong!

Hard as it may be to believe, Jessica once tipped the scales at 170 pounds. She tried various diets, exercise plans, motivational programs— you name it, she tried it—but nothing worked. While some plans seemed to work at first, the success was always short-lived. She'd always gain the weight back and then some.

One day, after the latest uncomfortable argument with her mom about her size, Jessica decided to take a different approach. Instead of swallowing her feelings and frustrations along with a candy bar, she headed to her back porch and climbed aboard an old, rickety stationary bike. As she pushed down on the pedals for the first time, both the flywheel and her muscles groaned with rust and disuse. She told herself, *I will just do this for 10 minutes, and if I still want that candy bar afterward, I'll have it.*

While those 10 minutes were pretty rough, she felt great afterward— and she had lost the urge to dig into the chocolate. This experience was the start of a gradual shift for Jessica. Slowly but surely, she kept making small, incremental changes in her health routine. Eventually, she added a few more 10-minute bursts of activity throughout her day, until gradually she slimmed down successfully and permanently.

On the other hand, Liz had always stayed relatively thin by eating carefully and exercising like a maniac. Then she had a baby. Once she became a working mom, all of her free time suddenly vanished. She struggled daily to find a break in the action and had trouble squeezing in her usual workouts. Just getting out for a walk to stretch her legs became a luxury. Having a newborn also affected her sleep routine, and feeling lethargic, she began reaching for sugary, starchy foods to give her energy. Predictably, her weight started to creep up.

Realizing she had to do something or live with the excess baby weight, Liz decided to change her approach to exercise. Instead of looking to fit 60 minutes worth of exercise into a single block of time, she started doing several short, intense workouts throughout the day. She took up meditation to help manage stress, got a grip on her eating and sleep habits, and looked for ways to engineer movement back into her day whenever it was convenient. Soon she was back to her pre-baby weight.

Although we came to the same conclusion in different ways and for different reasons, we both experienced firsthand how effective the *Thin in 10* approach is for weight loss and fitness. Jessica remembers that first

10 minutes on her bike as one of her proudest accomplishments; it's the moment that started her journey to lighter weight and better health. She takes this experience to heart now that she's a fitness professional helping others who are at the very same crossroads where she herself once stood. Liz now understands that it isn't necessary to grind it out for hours on end to have the body you want.

Thin in 10 works because it addresses all three pillars of weight loss—diet, exercise, and lifestyle—in a way that's so quick and easy anyone can do it—including you. You have just read how well it worked for us. We're certain the *Thin in 10* approach works for everyone across the fitness spectrum—from people just starting on their journey toward a healthier, thinner life, to those who are fit but in need of some time management or food control skills. Best of all, regardless of how much you currently exercise or how well you eat, success comes almost *immediately* with this program. However, we can't emphasize enough that this is not a short-term quick fix; this is a program you can stick with the rest of your life. *Thin in 10* is about creating a lasting, lifestyle change that helps you lose and maintain your weight loss for the long term.

Why Is Weight Loss So Elusive?

In theory, weight loss should be easy. You cut back a little on the calories, spend an hour at the gym three to four times a week, and the pounds should peel off. Right? Wrong. Even celebrities with more than enough money, help, and resources often struggle to lose excess weight. If they can't make it happen, how can the rest of us? Why is it so hard to shrink yourself down to proper size and stay there?

Research subjects who drastically cut back on calories while dramatically increasing their activity do absolutely lose weight over the course of the eight- to twenty-four-week study. Unfortunately, what happens in the lab doesn't always translate to the real world. And, of course, we don't usually find out what happens in the months and years after the scientists pack up their clipboards, scales, and fat-measuring tools, leaving the subjects to their own devices. The few reports on long-term follow-up that do exist show most participants in weight-loss studies regain all the weight over time.

This is also true of contestants on the reality show *Biggest Loser*. As the television season progresses, almost all of the contestants drop a significant number of pounds—and quickly. We root for them while they're on-screen but don't see everything they go through behind the scenes. Nor do we keep track of former contestants. Well here's some more reality for you: Fewer than half of all former *Biggest Loser* contestants maintain their weight loss (only time will tell if this percentage shrinks further).

The truth is, without a team of scientists or a screaming personal trainer standing over you, counting every morsel you consume and cheering you on each time you step on the treadmill, it's nearly impossible to stick with a plan forever, especially if that plan is unreasonable, restrictive, or uncomfortable (as most popular diet and exercise programs are).

Many weight-loss systems ask for *a lot* of effort on your part and then don't deliver much in return. Do you want to give up your favorite foods forever? Can you spare an hour or more every single day to devote to exercise? No? Then inevitably you'll "slip up" because you feel starved, cheated, and overworked.

That's where we come in. Our *Thin in 10* approach is different. It isn't about depriving yourself, making your workouts a chore, or striving to attain some fantasy, manipulated image. It's not about eating this and avoiding that. We don't demand that you spin, step, or run yourself into the ground or stop eating chocolate. Rather, this program is about making exercise and good nutrition work for you and fitting it into your already overscheduled daily routine—day in and day out, year after year. Simple changes executed 10 minutes at a time. That's the best way to achieve lasting weight-loss success.

Why It Works

Many health organizations offer guidelines for getting into shape and losing weight. For example, the American College of Sports Medicine recommends 30 minutes of moderate activity each day to increase stamina and lower the risk of heart disease. The Institutes of Medicine advises at least an hour of moderate activity a day for optimal health benefits and weight maintenance and up to 90 minutes a day for weight loss.

All of these recommendations are well intentioned and accurate. We in no way wish to criticize expert medical guidelines. However, none of these takes into account how hard it is for so many people to take the first step.

Thin in 10 gets you moving down the road toward success 10 minutes at a time. It's a realistic and sustainable approach that helps you lose weight and, more important, keep it off. You don't have to take our word for it. The *Thin in 10* concept—sometimes dubbed "exercise snacking" by experts—has been shown to be just as, or even more, effective than the long, slow-burn approach. Studies dating back more than a decade have found that 10-minute workout sessions can be helpful for both losing and maintaining weight. This growing body of research started with a ground-breaking investigation by the University of Pittsburg, which concluded that mini-workout sessions are so productive they could prevent obesity.[1]

More recently, Canadian researchers concluded that short, intense workouts are possibly more effective for weight loss than long, drawn-out slow workouts. They even remarked that one really good, intense short workout can produce the same caloric burn and cardiovascular benefits as a long but leisurely paced workout.[2] A 2010 Massachusetts General Hospital study found that 10 minutes of exercise taps into both stored and blood-borne fats, which helps with weight loss and maintenance and improves overall health.[3] And a Norwegian study conducted just recently discovered that shorter bouts of exercise can be just as effective for fitness and weight loss as longer ones, provided the exercise is intense enough and done on a regular basis.[4]

Besides the research conclusions and our personal experiences, we held a focus group to see which of our diet, exercise, and lifestyle strategies work best. While our work with the focus group wasn't a scientific endeavor, it helped us work out the kinks of our program and understand general preferences. Our group was comprised of fifty women between the ages of twenty-five and sixty-five who came in all shapes and sizes and with a variety of schedules. They followed the *Thin in 10* approach for twelve weeks. Believe us when we tell you they were vocal about what they liked and didn't like about the program.

Based on the group's feedback, we refined the original program. In the end, their consensus was that *Thin in 10* works because it's sustainable. It's a manageable plan they were able to follow right from the get-go, and it helped them make huge leaps toward their weight-loss goals without feeling overwhelmed by a bunch of restrictive rules. What's more, by the time the twelve-week pilot ended, nearly all of our participants had begun to see changes in their bodies and weight and asked to continue the program. The results, even if short term, are promising. Many of our testers have been able to maintain their weight loss and attribute this to the ease of making these 10-minute changes a part of their lives. As one focus group member, Ronit, put it, "It is simply a part of my daily living and so doesn't feel like a program anymore." Another member, Christina, wrote in her follow-up evaluation, "The program helped me get my motivation back on track. By committing to the 10 minutes of exercise, it helped because I knew I could do the 10 minutes but I usually was so energized and into it that I would go longer. I am exercising at least five days a week now. I also really enjoyed the 10-minute walk and like to keep that incorporated especially after dinner. I am doing better on my eating and have lost more weight."

We thank all our focus group participants for their dedication and hard work. The plan wouldn't be as solid or as user-friendly without them. And by the way, it's not too late to join the *Thin in 10* family! Join us online at www.thinin10.com and share your story with us. We've got tons of extra information, giveaways (to help you stay motivated), resources, additional workouts, recipes, and a community to help you achieve your goals. You can even log on and ask us questions about the plan.

The *Thin in 10* Program

The *Thin in 10* program consists of three pillars, or segments. Part 1 focuses on exercise, part 2 focuses on diet, and part 3 focuses on lifestyle. Each of these three areas is equally important in achieving your weight-loss and healthy-living goals.

Five 10-minute workouts form the core of part I and the *Thin in 10* program. We've carefully designed each workout to use your body in a different way so you get the most from your session. Chapter 1, "Your 10-Minute Exercise Plan," includes a detailed description of where to begin based on your fitness level, how to progress, and the kind of results you can expect. We've designed our routines so that no matter where you're starting, you can get going and make adjustments, as needed. For example, if you're just new to exercise and would classify yourself as a couch potato, follow the "Get Started" plan, which gradually ramps up by slowly increasing the intensity and frequency of your workouts (no need to overdo it at first as you do with some programs).

Perhaps you're already exercising above and beyond what we recommend in the plan. If so, don't stop what you're doing! One way to incorporate the *Thin in 10* workouts into your current routine is by tacking on the extra 10 minutes at the beginning or end of what you already do. You'll barely notice an extra 10 minutes here or there in your workouts but adding these minutes pushes you just an extra little bit. Another way to work the plan is to cut back your current routine and make up the lost time with the *Thin in 10* workouts. Either way, these routines can be easily integrated into your workout schedule.

Whatever level you're currently at, only the Total Body Circuit workout requires exercise equipment—a resistance band. But if you don't have a band, no worries. We've got alternative options for you (more about this in chapter 5). You simply use your body as resistance when you do the other routines. There's no need to fuss with a bunch of clunky chunks of iron or with exercise balls rolling out from under you during any of the workouts. However, since each workout is just 10 minutes, don't expect any of them to be a walk in the park, even the walking routines. When you're only exercising for 10 minutes at a time, we ask you to give a full-throttle effort to be rewarded with maximum calorie burn and sculpting power.

Also, if you're looking for a bonus workout or a change of pace, by all means pop the DVD into the player and use those workouts. The DVD doubles your choices; they are completely different workouts than the ones featured in the book yet they complement the book's workouts perfectly. You can swap workouts as follows:

Book	DVD
Core & More	Core Conditioning
Cardio QUICK	Cardio Quickie
Simple Strength	Strength Shot
The 10-Minute Total Body Circuit	Total Body Band
The 10-Minute Stretch	Stretch & De-stress

In part II, the meal plan is structured to make eating for weight loss a straightforward operation. Rather than putting you on another "diet," we consulted with a registered dietitian to develop the simplest way to eat healthy and make your meals quickly. Because we believe that food is more than just the sum of its chemical parts, the plan isn't based on manipulating carbohydrates, fat, or any other nutrient. Instead, it's based on enjoying the foods you love in moderation. Eating in a way that makes you feel happy and satisfied is the best way to prevent going overboard on calories.

There's no complicated math or calorie counting to contend with either. Each recipe has been created to stay within the calorie limits we've set for each meal: 300 for breakfast, 400 for lunch, 600 for dinner, and a discretionary 200 for snacks, desserts, and beverages. Following the menus, suggestions, and recipes gives you between 1,300 and 1,500 calories of food a day. For most women, that's enough that they don't feel starved yet are still able to lose weight. If you are exercising beyond the amount the plan lays out, you may need to up your calorie intake but we caution you not to get into an "earn and burn" mentality where you use exercise to rationalize overeating and poor food choices. And focusing on whole, unprocessed foods (like the ones we've included in the plan) helps curb hunger. Men may need to increase portion sizes or add an extra snack to reach 1,800 calories if they feel too hungry when following the plan.

The meal plan adheres to the *Thin in 10* philosophy: You don't need to be a whiz in the kitchen to make any of these meals in 10 minutes or less. And yes, we tested them all to make sure they really are that easy and fast to prepare.

Finally, in part III, we offer ways to improve your results, boost your energy, and enhance your overall health. In this section, we explain things like how moving more during the day, getting a good night's sleep, and having a strategy to get you through a period of low motivation can speed up weight loss.

So, what do you think? Isn't it time you start losing weight and get the body you have always dreamed of . . . for good? Surely you can carve out 10 minutes at a time to move toward your goals and realize your full potential. This is the plan that's going to work for you once and for all. We'll be with you every step of the way. Let's get started!

Pay Attention to These Sections

Throughout this book, you'll occasionally see highlighted sections we want you to pay extra attention to. Keep your eyes peeled for the following four special sections:

(S) implify It:

This section appears next to the easier versions of an exercise in chapters 2–7. These are the moves to try if you find the basic version of the routine a little too challenging.

(A) dvance It:

When you're ready to push yourself a bit harder than the basic version of an exercise found in chapters 2–7, scan the page for this section to learn how.

The *Thin in 10* Advantage As if you need any more reasons to do this plan, this section points out one of the plan's special benefits; often this is a benefit that is not obvious so we want to make sure you know about it.

RD Recommendation RD is short for "registered dietitian." This marker appears in chapters 9–11. It highlights recommendations and easy-to-follow tips related to the diet plan.

The *Thin in 10* Exercise Plan

CHAPTER

1

Your 10-Minute Exercise Plan

The *Thin in 10* program proves once and for all that you do have time to work out. Getting fit, feeling good, and losing weight doesn't mean laboring for hours in a gym or spending hundreds of dollars on bulky high-tech equipment. The *Thin in 10* workouts are so concentrated, they get the job done 10 minutes at a time and require little or no equipment. You will be able to fit fitness into your life on a regular, consistent basis.

Whether you've been exercising for years or are just starting out, the next six chapters in part I outline a balanced, efficient weekly routine that is right for you. The routines hit all aspects of a complete fitness program: cardio calorie burning, strength and sculpt, flexibility and balance, and core and posture. Putting them all together gives you a time-compacted routine that's manageable and effective.

Here's How It Works

Before beginning your workout program, it's important to determine the starting point that's right for you. To do this, spend a few moments taking the following brief fitness quiz. Retake the quiz every four to six weeks to determine if you're ready to move on to the next level. Chances are you will already know this by how you feel, but retake the quiz to confirm your decision. We also recommend taking a few moments to set your goals. (See "Setting SMART Goals" on page 22.)

Once you've determined your current fitness level, commit to your workout times and mark them on your calendar. Spend some time learning the routines provided for your fitness level. For example, beginners start with the walking program only, while advanced exercisers include all five workouts in their weekly schedule from the get-go.

Determining Your Starting Point

We can't emphasize enough the importance of getting your doctor's clearance before starting this or any other exercise program. This is especially true if you have medical issues, have had medical issues in the past, or haven't exercised since bell-bottoms were in style—the first time around. Checking in with your doctor helps you stay safe and get the most from your program.

Your Starting Point Quiz

For each question, circle the answer that best reflects your situation; then add up how many *a*, *b*, *c*, or *d* responses you circled to determine your score. Plan on retaking this quiz every four to six weeks as your fitness level improves.

1. *Which best describes your current workout routine?*
   a. It's been six months or more since I have exercised.
   b. I've been exercising, but sporadically—not more than three to four times a month.
   c. I've exercised at least three days a week for the past six months.
   d. I exercise most days of the week and do both endurance and resistance training.

2. *Which option below best describes your current endurance level?*
   a. It's tough for me to walk at a moderate pace for more than 10 minutes at a time.
   b. I can walk at a moderate pace for more than 20 continuous minutes without getting winded.
   c. I can run or walk very quickly for 30 minutes or more without feeling fatigued.
   d. I can easily complete 45–60 minutes of moderate- to high-intensity aerobic activity.

3. *When you're pushing yourself hard in a workout, how do you feel?*
   a. Like I can barely finish.
   b. Pathetic and out of shape.
   c. Tired but determined.
   d. Fit and strong.

4. *Which option below best describes your current strength level?*
   a. I haven't done any strength or resistance training in the past 30 days.
   b. I have a little experience lifting weights and performing resistance exercises.

Your Starting Point Quiz   continued

c. I do strength or resistance training at least two days a week.

d. I do strength or resistance training three days a week or more.

5. *What would happen if you attempted a push-up?*
a. Forget it. My arms would collapse!
b. I can do a push-up from my knees.
c. I can probably eke out one full push-up on my toes.
d. I can do at least two full push-ups.

6. *What would happen if you attempted to do abdominal crunches?*
a. I couldn't do one without a struggle.
b. I can manage a few of them.
c. I can do at least fifteen but would be sore the next day.
d. I can do at least two sets of fifteen crunches with ease.

7. *Which best describes you?*
a. I have quite a lot of weight to lose.
b. I could lose some weight.
c. I am at or near my ideal weight but could use some toning up.
d. I'm at or near my ideal weight and my body is toned.

Now review your answers to questions 1–7. Next to each letter, write down how many times you answered a question with that response.

a. _____

b. _____

c. _____

d. _____

Answer Key

If more of your answers are *a*, start with our GET STARTED plan.

If more of your answers are *b*, start with our NOVICE plan.

If more of your answers are *c*, start with our INTERMEDIATE plan.

If more of your answers are *d*, start with our ADVANCED plan.

If your answers are nearly evenly split between two or more letters, choose the letter that represents the least advanced workout schedule.

Weekly Recommendations

Wherever you are on the fitness spectrum, once you're ready to start the *Thin in 10* workouts, we ask that you use the following weekly workout schedule based on your current fitness level. The fitter you are, the more sessions you can add—but we'll never ask you to do more than 10 minutes at a time or more than 40 minutes a day (and that's only at the advanced level).

> "Evaluate your progress every four to six weeks."

Evaluate your progress every four to six weeks. At that time, if you're ready for more, move up a level. If not, repeat the same workout schedule for another four to six weeks and then reevaluate. Go at your own pace. If you start out at the advanced level, don't worry. We've outlined numerous options to make the program more challenging without increasing your time commitment.

Read through the recommendations for each level to fully understand what's expected of you each week. Feel free to schedule your days as you wish; for example, your Day 1 can be a Sunday, Monday, or Tuesday. Select whatever works best for you and your schedule. If we ask you to repeat a session that same day, you can do them back-to-back, split them up into morning and evening sessions, or spread them out in any other way that works for you. We're giving you four options to choose from: Get Started, Novice, Intermediate, and Advanced. Choose which level works best for you right now and reevaluate your fitness every four to six weeks.

Get Started Plan

Up to 20 minutes, 7 days a week

What is your goal? Just to get in the habit of moving! Don't think about this as "exercise." Simply focus on getting your body in motion every day. Newbies and novices start out with the walking program, walking at a level 1 intensity (see page 29). You may move up to level 2 walking intensity (see page 31) by the fourth week, but it's okay if you don't. It's also okay if at first you can't complete the full 10 minutes all at once. Just do what you can and build from there. Getting started is a victory in and of itself.

Can't walk outdoors? Set your timer and walk laps around your house, the mall, or an indoor track. March in place. No excuses! This is a *must-do* every day. You'll add in your stretching routine in week 3 of the program.

After four to six weeks, reevaluate your fitness level. Do you feel stronger? Do you have more endurance? Did the answers to Your Starting Point Quiz change? If you're ready for more, move up to the next level, the Novice plan. If you're not, stay right where you are for another four to six weeks; then reevaluate.

Day	Thin in 10 Workouts	Total Time (minutes)
1	Level 1 Walk	10
2	Level 1 Walk	10
3	Level 1 Walk	
	Stretch	20
	(add in week 3 of program)	
4	Level 1 Walk	10
5	Level 1 Walk	10
6	Level 1 Walk	10
7	Level 1 Walk	
	Stretch	20
	(add in week 3 of program)	

Novice Plan

Up to 20 minutes, 7 days a week

The Novice plan asks for the same commitment to walking as the Get Started plan: 10 minutes, seven days a week. The big difference is that this level asks for a bit more effort, intensity, and form and adds in several more of the workout programs. Also, your total daily commitment is up to 20 minutes. Do your sessions all at once or split them up into 10-minute bursts of activity throughout the day. For example, most people start out this program doing a level 1 or 2 walking style but may move up to level 3 by the end of week 4 (see page 32).

After four to six weeks, reevaluate your fitness level. Do you feel stronger? Do you have more endurance? Did the answers to Your Starting Point Quiz change? If you're ready for more, move to the Intermediate plan. If you're not, stay right where you are for another four to six weeks and then reevaluate.

Day	Thin in 10 Workouts	Total Time (minutes)
1	Walk	
	Simple Strength	20
2	Walk	
	Core & More	20
3	Walk	
	Stretch	20
4	Walk	
	Cardio QUICK	20
5	Walk	10
6	Walk	
	Stretch	20
7	Walk	10

Intermediate Plan

Up to 30 minutes, 7 days a week

As with all other plans, walking seven days a week at the highest intensity you can handle is the foundation of the Intermediate plan. You will also integrate some of the other programs into your routine and work out up to 30 minutes a day. You can do all of your workouts at once or spread them out through the day. Do whatever works best with your schedule.

At this point, walking at level 2 or 3 (see pages 31–32) may be appropriate. You can consider moving up to level 4 walking (see page 34), which incorporates some running, but it isn't mandatory by any means. When you find that you're able to master the base moves, consider trying a few of our "Advance It" suggestions. After four to six weeks, reevaluate your fitness level. Do you feel stronger? Do you have more endurance? Did the answers to Your Starting Point Quiz change? If you're ready for more, move to the Advanced plan. If you're not, stay right where you are for another four to six weeks; then reevaluate.

Day	Thin in 10 Workouts	Total Time (minutes)
1	Walk	
	Simple Strength	
	Stretch	30
2	Walk	
	Cardio QUICK	
	Core & More	30
3	Walk	
	Total Body Circuit	
	Stretch	30
4	Walk	
	Cardio QUICK—2x	30
5	Walk	
	Simple Strength—2x	30
6	Walk	
	Total Body Circuit—2x	30
7	Walk	
	Stretch	20

Advanced Plan

Up to 40 minutes, 7 days a week

This plan calls for to 40 minutes of workouts per day and incorporates every single *Thin in 10* workout program. Following the Advanced plan usually involves walking at level 3 (see page 32). You can consider doing some of your walks at level 4 (see page 34), which involves short periods of running, but it isn't mandatory.

It's likely you're now ready to incorporate "Advance It" options on any or all of your moves. You'll be completing more sessions, which means more workout minutes per day. Sessions can still be split into mini workout sessions or done all at once, depending on your schedule.

Day	*Thin in 10* Workouts	Total Time (minutes)
1	Walk Simple Strength—2x Stretch (two split sessions, or in a row)	40
2	Walk Cardio QUICK—2x Core & More	40
3	Walk Total Body Circuit—2x Stretch (two split sessions, or in a row)	40
4	Walk Cardio QUICK—2x	30
5	Walk Simple Strength—2x (two split sessions, or in a row)	30
6	Walk Total Body Circuit—2x (two split sessions, or in a row).	30
7	Walk Stretch	20

Goal Setting: Deciding What You *Really* Want

Sure, weight loss is a great goal, but it can be a pretty empty and generic one. As you begin the *Thin in 10* plan, we encourage you to think beyond losing weight. For, example, if you'd like to be thirty pounds lighter than you are today, fitting into your skinny jeans is only part of what you're after. A good weight-loss plan is also a lifestyle plan, which ultimately includes feeling better and having more energy to do everything you want to pursue. The scale only tells part of the story.

It pays to pinpoint aspects of your goal that go beyond skin deep to help you stay inspired. For instance, did you know that a 2009 survey of 3,000 brides found that 22 percent of them packed on twenty-one pounds after the wedding? Most of the gain comes within the first year of marriage! And more evidence shows that married men and married women are more than twice as likely to become obese as single people. Most of the newlyweds interviewed cited lack of motivation as the reason for the weight gain. By focusing on developing *Thin in 10* habits that endure beyond the honeymoon, you can look like you do in your wedding pictures at your twentieth-anniversary party.

Setting SMART Goals

The best method of goal setting we've found is the SMART goal system—setting Specific, Measurable, Attainable, Realistic goals that are on a set Timetable.

Think of your SMART goals as a way of drawing a map from where you are now to where you want to be. Let's use losing weight as an example.

Specific
Saying you want to lose weight is a rather vague goal—kind of like saying you want to go to Disney World. Which park? Which hotel? When? With whom? You're better off selecting a concrete number, preferably based on real information such as body mass index (BMI), a doctor's recommendation, or an ideal weight chart.

Setting SMART Goals   continued

Measurable

Choose how to track your weight loss. You can measure pounds lost on a scale, but you could also measure inches or changes in BMI. Just choose a measurement or series of measurements that easily show your progress.

Attainable

You can achieve most any goal you set when you plan your steps wisely and establish a realistic time frame in which to carry out those steps. One way to make goals attainable is by taking your ultimate goal and breaking it up into smaller "stepping stone" goals. That way, goals don't seem too overwhelming, and you are in a state of perpetual success.

Realistic

Losing fifty pounds in two weeks? Not so realistic. Losing five pounds in two weeks? That's more reasonable. You set yourself up to feel like a failure if your goals are unrealistic.

Timely

So long as it's realistic, having a time frame in which you wish to accomplish your goals is a good idea. It gives you the sense that the clock is ticking and the ball is in motion. Instead of saying you'll do it "someday," get started now. Set some SMART goals.

Wrap-Up

As we've explained, the *Thin in 10* program is a simple, straightforward approach to losing weight and changing your life. We know you can do it! Now let's move on to your first program, The 10-Minute Walk, where we'll show you how to take the first steps toward your best body ever.

SMART Goal Setter

Now it's time to set some goals of your own using this SMART Goal Setter. You can create your own goal setter in your personal workout journal, make photocopies of this page, or visit www.thinin10.com to get your customizable goal worksheet.

Specific
_____
_____
_____
_____

Measurable
_____
_____
_____
_____

Attainable
_____
_____
_____
_____

Realistic
_____
_____
_____
_____

Timely
_____
_____
_____
_____

CHAPTER
2 | The 10-Minute
Walk

"This workout (like all the workouts) fits beautifully into my daily schedule and existing routine."
—Ilan, original *Thin in 10* focus group member

Walking is as basic a fitness activity as they come. It doesn't get any simpler than putting one foot in front of the other, wouldn't you agree? Don't let the ease of execution fool you though. When you learn to walk with purpose and intention, there's no better way to whip your heart, lungs, and muscles into shape, up endurance, lift your spirits, and yes, help shrink your body down to size. That's why the walking program is the first workout in your *Thin in 10* plan.

Why Walking Works!

We should tell you up front that walking doesn't exactly melt calories like butter on hot toast. Depending on the type of walking you do, you might burn just half the calories that you would in the high-intensity workouts described in the upcoming chapters. Yet, although walking isn't a calorie-burning inferno, we believe it's an essential element of your weight-loss plan. (And, as the plan progresses, we offer lots of tips on pumping up the calorie burn of your walking workouts.)

To begin with, there's no learning curve. Other than babies just hitting their milestone to get up and amble forth, most of us are already walking experts. Sure, we've got plenty of tips and tricks for you to make the most of your efforts, but mastering this workout begins by taking the very first step. You may have given up on other workouts right away because they made you feel clumsy, awkward, or silly. There's no such excuse with walking. Even if you've got creaky joints, you can probably start with at least a few minutes of walking at a time and slowly build up without undue pain or injury. In fact, exercise is often the best medicine for joint aches.

> "Exercise is often the best medicine for joint aches."

Here's another major advantage walking has over most other fitness activities: It doesn't require a lot of equipment. No helmets, gloves, wrenches, pumps, knee pads, wrist guards, caps, goggles, pools, or poles. Just lace up your shoes, open the front door, and off you go. Heading for the nearest treadmill works too. We do suggest a good pair of walking shoes and, for women, a decent bra (see page 33) to minimize the bounce, but you might already have these items in your closet. If you don't, see our walking shoes and gear advice on pages 36 and 37.

Of course, running is just as accessible and convenient as walking, but it isn't the best choice for many exercisers. For one thing, walking is considerably easier on your joints, tendons, and ligaments. While frequent injuries can be a real issue with high-impact activities like running, almost everyone has joints that can handle a walking program. In addition, most people are able to complete the entire walk routine the very first time they try it. Although some beginners may feel out of breath and wish they could bail, most people can walk for at least 10 minutes straight without feeling winded or achy. From there, it's fairly easy to build up stamina. Even if you're not ready for a full 10-minute stint at the get-go, it will happen. (For those who do like to run, we've given you an option for this at level 4, on page 34.)

That's just the short list of reasons for why we've made a daily walk the first workout routine in *Thin in 10*. The science we've looked at offers even more reasons. For example, a study published in the *Journal of the*

American Medical Association found that brisk walking is very effective for reducing deep abdominal fat—the most dangerous kind of fat, which pads your internal organs and produces hormones and other substances that can raise blood pressure, negatively alter good and bad cholesterol levels, and impair the body's ability to use insulin (insulin resistance). It's associated with a higher risk of heart disease, type 2 diabetes, cancer, and a host of other health maladies including premature death.[5]

A University of Colorado study found that when people commit to walking 10–15 minutes more than what they typically do in a day, they don't necessarily lose weight but they may stop gaining weight.[6] What's more, the majority of participants in the National Weight Control Registry, an ongoing survey of more than 3,000 people who have lost at least thirty pounds and kept it off for more than a year, report walking as their number one exercise strategy for losing weight and keeping it off.

Your 10-Minute Walking Program

Before you start your walking program, read through the various levels of walking that we've created for the program to determine your appropriate starting point. It's important to select the level that pushes you to work but not so hard that you feel sore and discouraged after a workout. Also consider which program it's wise to start with. For example, if you haven't exercised in a while, it's probably best to start with the Getting Started program and level 1 walking. Likewise, if you're a more experienced exerciser and walking is not problematic for you, level 3 or 4 is more likely your speed.

In keeping with the idea of simplicity, you're going to do a 10-minute walk every day. Use the first minute to heat up your body and get your muscles into the groove;

> "You can do your walk program at any time of day."

for a basic 10-minute walk, 1 minute should be all the warm-up that's needed. After the first minute, gradually increase your speed and intensity until you are walking at the ideal pace and style for your level of walking; continue that pace for the next 9 minutes. That's it. Really.

You can do your walk program at any time of day. Because you're only doing 10 minutes, it isn't necessary to suit up into workout gear. Just slip on a decent pair of walking shoes and go. You can build your 10-minute walk into your day as a commute to work, a lunchtime break, a pre-dinner pick-me-up, or any time in between—even walking in place counts. Seriously consider using it as a post-dinner ritual: One study found that walking immediately after a meal helped subjects lose more weight than if they walked an hour after eating.[7] Plus, it's a great way to avoid heading straight to the couch in the evening. But no matter when you decide to do it, the most important part of this program is to be consistent and skip as few of the workouts as possible.

We've assumed that most readers are just starting an exercise program and will begin with our easy 10-minute plans. However, if you're already doing a regular workout, add in the 10-minute walk anyway. Consider it a bonus. As we said in the intro, incorporating the *Thin in 10* program into a program you've already started is perfectly doable and helps you reach your goals more quickly.

Find Your Level

Another important advantage to walking is that it can be easily adapted—as your fitness improves, you can easily do more; in this way, the workout grows with you. Beginners start with the level 1 walk style and then gradually progress to the advanced level 3 walk style. There's also an optional level 4 for those who want to move on to a different type of challenge, but if your body isn't built for high impact, you can hold steady at level 3 and still get an amazing workout. The beauty of this approach is the workouts progress and continue to provide results without you necessarily increasing the amount of time you devote to them.

10-MINUTE WALK WORKOUT

Keep in Mind
- choose the level of walking that suits your current condition and preferences
- aim to do the 10-minute walk workout every day or at least most days of the week

What You Need
- good pair of walking shoes (recommended)
- sports bra (optional)

What to Expect
- a highly variable calorie burn that depends on level of walking style, speed, distance, and body weight
- to develop (or reinforce) the habit of daily exercise

Here's a rundown on the four different walking levels, along with information on choosing your starting point and determining when you're ready to progress:

Level 1

Level 1 is the easiest walking style. It's similar to just walking down the street or through the mall, except that you pay more attention to posture, gait, and intensity. Expect to move at an average pace of 20 minutes a mile; in other words, you can cover about half a mile in 10 minutes. You'll burn about forty calories in that time, depending on factors such as your body weight and metabolism. The primary muscles that get a workout at this level are calves, thighs, hips, and core. Stamina and muscular endurance increase as you prepare to move up to level 2.

Choose level 1 if you haven't exercised in recent memory or if even a few minutes of physical activity leaves you breathless and tired. This might also be a good place to start if you have chronic joint issues such as stiff knees or a temperamental back. Check with your doctor before you start this program.

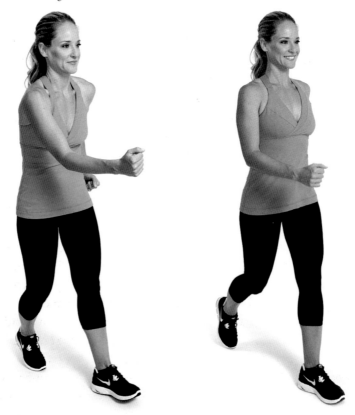

Technique: Walk at a comfortable pace with a taller posture than you would usually have when going on a casual stroll.

- Lift and open your chest. Keep your head up and centered between your shoulders, with your shoulders relaxed, back, and down. It should feel like your head and neck are floating effortlessly between your shoulders.
- Keep your arms low and slightly bent, and as you move, swing them naturally and easily. Your hands should be cupped gently rather than open or squeezed into fists. Tighten the core muscles of your abdominals and lower back ever so slightly to reinforce the feeling of tallness.
- As you move, think of powering from your hips rather than your thighs. Your stride should feel unforced but a bit longer and more purposeful than usual.
- As for your feet, roll heel-arch-ball-toe before completing the step and moving into the next one.

Move up a level when you can do the entire 10-Minute Walk workout in the level 1 walking style for at least three days in a row without feeling winded or sore. You always have the option to stay right here. Consistently getting out and moving is what produces results. However, moving up a level burns more calories and tones more muscles. You have the option of walking at level 1 on some days and at a higher level on others if you feel you can't make the jump up in intensity all at once.

Level 2

At level 2, you pick up the pace to burn more calories and get a more strenuous cardio workout. Most people walking at level 2 move at a brisk pace of three and a half to four miles an hour, so in 10 minutes they cover somewhere around six-tenths of a mile and burn about fifty calories. The extra effort and calorie burn is partly due to the faster pace and covering more distance in less time, but it's also the result of the posture and technique involved. At this level, you use your hips and buttocks even more than in level 1 and your arm swing is more powerful too. This contributes to increased calorie burning—and toning potential for virtually every muscle in your body.

Choose level 2 if the walking workout at level 1 is a no-brain-no-painer, and you are ready for more. If you've been working out on a regular basis for at least three months and you don't have any chronic joint complaints yet you're not quite ready to charge ahead with all cylinders firing, this is the right level of walking for you.

Technique: Walking tall is every bit as important in level 2 as in level 1.

- Keep your chest lifted; your head, neck, and shoulders relaxed; and your core tight. Don't squeeze those hands into fists either.
- Walk at a pace that's significantly faster and more intense than your level 1 pace.
- Bend your arms 90 degrees and pump them with determination as you walk. Swing them back and forth—not side to side—and keep them close to your body. At the top of the arm swing, your elbow should be level with your breastbone; at the bottom of the arm swing, your hand brushes your hip.
- Take shorter, faster strides that once again power from the hips while keeping your hips loose and in a natural position.
- Land firmly on your heel and roll smoothly to push off with your

toes. Think of planting your heel and then pushing the ground away from you as you roll through your foot.

- Focus on intensity gauges like breathing and heart rate too: Your breathing should be audible but steady and in control, and your heart should be thumping but not pounding out of your chest.

Move up a level when you can do the entire 10-Minute Walk workout in the level 2 walking style for at least three days in a row without feeling winded or sore. You always have the option to stay right here or to mix and match your levels to suit your needs. As you add in the other workouts to your program, you may find yourself dropping back to level 1 for a while or at least some of the days. That's okay. But when you're ready, do move on to level 3 on at least some days. The more effort you put into your workout, the better your results.

Level 3

People doing a level 3 walk resemble race walkers with a narrow stride, wiggling hips, and powerful arm swing. Walking at the lightning-quick pace of about five miles per hour allows you to scorch through about eight-tenths of a mile in 10 minutes. Some joggers move at about the same speed and that's the secret behind the success that comes with level 3 walking—it's an amazing workout for toning muscles and melting fat. Scientists speculate that walking so fast that you have to hold yourself back from running burns one and a half to two times the calories as walking at a slower pace—about sixty to eighty calories in 10 minutes. That's because it takes a lot of energy and body muscle mass to resist breaking into a run and maintain a walking stride.

This is your level if you're in top shape and work out on a regular basis now without any recurring aches, pains, or soreness. You're ready to hit it hard and push yourself right to the edge of your comfort zone during your walks.

Technique: Your instinct may be to lengthen your stride when you try to speed up, but it's actually faster and more efficient to take more steps per minute at a stride that's slightly shorter than normal.

- Imagine you are walking along a tightrope where one stride must line up directly in front of another so you don't fall off.

- Your posture is still tall and relaxed, but because your stride is quick and linear, your hips move from side to side in a sort of exaggerated cartoon wiggle.
- As you extend the forward leg, your knee stays fairly straight as your foot contacts the ground and bends only when you are about to swing your other leg forward.
- Each time you step, your fall lands square on the line directly in front of you so you don't stray from your imaginary tightrope.

Bra Basics

For women, any bra that allows you to walk without bouncing all over the place is fine for walking. It doesn't have to be an official sports bra either. However, you may prefer to wear a bra specifically designed for movement. We know some women who wear them all the time because they tend to be so comfortable. And if you choose carefully, you can even find one that gives you a complimentary silhouette under your regular clothes.

Sports bras come in two general types:

Compression bras have one chamber and press and flatten the breasts up against the chest as a single mass. Larger-breasted women may experience discomfort with this type of bra because the breasts may still bounce around as a single unit.

Encapsulation bras hold each breast in a separate cup so they stay in place and don't press against each other. Many of these bras are sized like traditional bras up to size DD, whereas compression bras usually come in small, medium, large, and extra-large.

Try both types to see which one works best for you. When you try on a sports bra, raise your arms over your head. If the elastic band at the bottom rises up, the bra is the wrong size for you. Try the next size up. Also, jump around in the dressing room. If your girls bounce there, they're definitely going to wiggle and jiggle when you walk! And make sure any exercise bra you consider is at least 25 percent Lycra for good stretch and hold.

A decent bra shouldn't set you back more than $20—far less if you shop the discounts and sales. Stretch the lifespan by hand-washing and air-drying bras whenever possible.

- Get a good toe lift by using your ankles. Land heel-first, roll through the foot, and then push off firmly and vigorously.
- Allow your legs to follow your arms. In other words, use your arms to propel your body forward and match your footfall to the rhythm of your arm swing.
- At this pace, you should be breathing pretty heavily and feeling your heart pounding by the end of the workout.

Structure your program: You may be up for the intensity of a level 3 walk daily or you might toss in a level 3 walk workout once a week to wake yourself up and burn a ton of calories. Feel free to mix and match levels however it suits you. Once you add in your other *Thin in 10* workouts, you might have to drop back a level on at least some of the days if you feel like you're overtraining. You do want to push yourself but always listen to your body.

Consider trying level 4 walk/run workouts if you are ready for more and you have no significant joint issues. Level 4 is a totally optional advancement for those who feel it would make their workouts more interesting. You don't need to go there to achieve your goals. We've already built in plenty of high-intensity, high-calorie-burning workouts into your *Thin in 10* program. You want to push yourself to your fullest potential, but the name of the game is consistency. If you tend to get injured when you run or if you find even small increments of running to be too much for your body, stick with the first three levels. Getting out there every day and moving on a regular basis is going to take you a lot further than doing one all-out routine that hurts you, bores you, or gives you an excuse to skip future workouts.

Level 4 (Optional)

By sprinkling running intervals throughout your walking workout, you can spike up exercise intensity and burn a few more calories than walking at the first two levels. The distance traveled at this level is about the same distance covered when walking at a level 3 pace, and the calorie burn is roughly equivalent as well, depending on your running speed. Try a level 4 workout if you think running might be an activity you'd enjoy. However, remember that this is an *optional* workout. You don't ever have to take a single running step if you don't want to or if it's not right for your body.

Try level 4 if you can do at least two level 3 walks per week without any recurring aches, pains, or soreness; you don't have a history of chronic joint problems; and you'd like to try some jogging for variety or if you're currently a jogger. This is a good workout for anyone who wants to spice up their walking routine without dramatically upping their risk of injury.

Technique: Start with 2 minutes of level 2 style walking; then alternate 1 minute of running at a moderate pace with 1 minute of walking at a level 2 pace for the remaining 8 minutes.

When you run, many of the same "stay tall and relaxed" posture reminders you use for walking are still important:

- Keep your head and chest lifted and your shoulders back and down.
- Gently pull your core inward. Your hands should be cupped into loose, relaxed fists.
- Bend your arms to slightly less than 90 degrees, and swing them back and forth while keeping them close to your body. At the

> "Focus on matching the rhythm of your breaths to your footfall."

  top of the arm swing, your elbow should be level with your breastbone; at the bottom of the swing, your hand brushes your hip.
- As with walking, your stride is powered from the hips, but here you need to drive your front knee up and forward as you extend your back leg to slightly lengthen your stride. It should almost feel as if you are falling forward as you run, so it feels slightly different from walking with tall posture. With your running stride, you can allow your upper body to slightly lean into your run.

When you run, your breathing should be deep and steady. Focus on matching the rhythm of your breaths to your footfall. Push yourself to the point that your heart is pounding evenly but not so hard that you feel like you're gargling your heart in your throat.

Pay attention to how you hold your body as you transition between walking and running. That's the point where your form is the most likely to fall apart. As you move between gaits, resist the urge to collapse in and downward or swing your arms across your body—these are the two most common transition mistakes we see. If you pay attention, they're easy enough to avoid or at least correct. Also, don't just stop. Keep moving the entire time. If you find you're too winded by the run portion to avoid stopping, switch back to level 2 or 3 and continue your walking workout schedule for a few more weeks; then try again.

Walking Gear Options

Again, you don't need any equipment to make a walk beneficial for exercise. However, if you are interested in any gadgets or gear to boost the power of your walks, we do have a few suggestions on what to try and what to skip:

Try: Walking poles. These trekking aids resemble ski poles and can be found in outdoor equipment specialty stores and on the Internet. Walking with poles—often called Nordic walking—increases the calorie burn of your walks by up to 40 percent. By gripping the handles and using the poles to push off the ground as you stride, you incorporate more upper-body muscles into your walk without adding any excess stress or strain on your joints. These poles can also be helpful if you have any lower-body joint issues or arthritis, as they may ease some of the stress on your knees or hips.

Skip: Holding dumbbells. Walkers often think that lugging around a pair of dumbbells is a great way to boost calorie burn and maybe add a little toning to their walks. The trouble is, swinging dumbbells can affect your natural stride and put extra stress on your joints, not your muscles (where you want it for toning purposes). If you want to add weight to your walk, consider a weighted vest instead (see below).

Try: Weighted vests. If your goal is to burn more calories, a weighted vest can be an effective and safe way to do it. Much like it sounds, a weighted vest drapes over your shoulders and wraps around your midsection. You can find weighted vests online or in most athletic stores; they are generally priced between $25 and $40, depending on the size and weight. A vest typically adds between two and sixteen pounds of extra weight where your body can handle it (and where most of us carry a little extra weight already)—at your core.

Skip: Ankle or wrist weights. Similar to dumbbells, these add extra weight to your body where it's hardest on your joints, increasing your risk for injury or strain.

What Shoe Is Right for You?

The risk of getting an overuse injury from walking is pretty low. You can reduce it further by wearing footwear designed for walking. The right footwear enhances comfort and makes walking more enjoyable too.

To choose a walking shoe, start by determining your walking pattern. Look at the bottom of an old pair of shoes; any type of shoe will do. Try to discover whether you are a pronator, a supinator, or are neutral (somewhere in the middle of the other foot strike patterns). If the wear is mainly to the inside edges of the shoe bottom, you're a *pronator*—you roll your foot inward as you walk. (Most women are pronators.) If the wear is mainly on the outside edges, you're a *supinator*—you strike down hardest on the outside of your foot. Both of these wear patterns, if extreme, can lead to sore ankles and knees.

Pronators should buy shoes with a motion-control device in the *midsole*, shoe-speak for the squishy center of the shoe between the part that encases your foot (the upper) and the part that touches the ground (the outsole). Look for a board-lasted shoe with the inside is glued rather than stitched in place. A straighter shoe with very little curve at the bottom is also preferable, as it provides additional support for the inside of the foot. Avoid overly padded models that feel squishy when you step, as they can exaggerate pronation.

Supinators should buy shoes with midsoles designed for extra shock absorbency and stability. Since supinators tend to have stiffer, less flexible feet, with inserts stitched into the bottom to keep the foot in place are a good choice. A shoe that has an inwardly curved shape is also suited to supinators. An extra bit of cushioning under the ball of the foot can help increase comfort, as long as the shoe doesn't cross the line into mushy.

A small percentage of people have "neutral feet" that don't roll excessively inward or outward. If you own this type of foot, you can wear just about any walking shoe. But even if your feet are absent of issues and you aren't especially injury prone, don't skimp on the basic walking shoe features. These include good shock absorption in the heels and in the balls of the feet and a very flexible forefoot that allows for the natural bend of the foot as you stride. The midsoles should be

What Shoe Is Right for You? continued

thinner than those of running shoes to accommodate a walking gait's slower foot roll, and the heels should be beveled, or slightly angled, to allow for a smooth heel-to-toe roll.

The great news here is that you don't need to plunk down a hundred dollars or more for a decent pair of walking shoes. We've found many shoes with all the features you need in the $20–$30 range; plus there are bargains to be had if you watch the sales and shop online. You can also find walking shoes that disguise themselves as dressier footwear—perfect if you tend to get your walks in during the workday. One tip for first-time buyers: Go to a shoe specialty shop and get a fitting by an expert. You can often still catch some sales; plus, once you find a model you like, you can hunt the Internet and box stores for a shoe that's the same or similar.

Wrap-Up

Both Liz and Jessica are avid walkers. Whatever else we do, both of us commit to a daily 10-minute walk. Our initial focus group members embraced the daily 10-minute walk as a terrific starting point to the program. We're confident you will too. Get started and see how easy it is to weave this workout into your life. You simply need a pair of comfy shoes—you don't need to change into workout gear, head for the gym, or do anything special. Ready, set. Go.

CHAPTER

3

Cardio
QUICK

"The cardio QUICK is one of my go-to
workouts to get me moving."
—Rebecca, original *Thin in 10* focus group member

I f you're looking for fast results, building some high-intensity cardio into your workouts is essential. Stacks of studies support this theory. For example, a recent Canadian study found that exercisers who completed a high-intensity interval training workout over a two-week period were much more effective at burning fat and carbohydrates both during and after exercise.[8] Other investigations into high-intensity training reported fat burning was greater compared with long, slow, and steady exercise and that two and a half hours of sweating it in high gear offered calorie and fat burn equal to ten and a half hours of long, slow distance training.[9] That said, high-intensity workouts can cause trouble too, by increasing your chances of injury, burnout, and overtraining. To get and maintain the best results, strike a balance between high- and low-intensity to shed pounds and pump up fitness—without sidelining yourself with sore joints and pulled muscles.

That's where interval-style training comes in. In fitness-speak, *interval training* means mixing spurts of high-intensity exercise with "rest periods" of lower-intensity exercise within the same workout session. Doing this gives you the best of both worlds: a boosted calorie burn and improved fitness level but a lowered risk of flaming out or limping off. You get a lot in return for your harder pushes, and since you allow your body to recover between efforts, you can last a lot longer without feeling completely destroyed.

Working out this way offers numerous other advantages too: If you're short on time for exercising, intervals allow you to trim back your time commitment without sacrificing results. Interval training has been shown to amp up the body's production of adrenaline, a hormone that helps reduce thigh and belly fat, two typical trouble zones. Some studies show high-intensity interval training is more effective for overall fat and weight loss even though the primary fuel burned during interval exercise is carbohydrate.

Fat versus Calories

True or false? Burning a higher percentage of fat during your workout is the best way to lose weight. The answer is false! You do burn a greater percentage of calories from fat (as opposed to carbohydrates) when you exercise slow and easy, but what matters most for weight loss is the total number of calories you burn. Walking at a leisurely pace for 10 minutes burns perhaps sixty calories; if you pick up the pace several notches, you can double that number. Even if the percentage of fat you burn is higher in the first workout, the second burns both more fat and more calories. So, go for the burn during the workout—the calorie burn, that is.

Intensity Deciphered

One of the most straightforward ways to track your exercise efforts is by using a Rate of Perceived Exertion (RPE) scale. You're your own best coach when it comes to knowing your exercise comfort zone. So ask yourself, *"How hard am I working right now?"* by referring to the RPE chart. For the 40-second low-intensity intervals, aim for a 5–6 RPE; for the 20-second high-intensity intervals, aim for an 8–9.

RPE Chart

Level	RPE	Test It
Easy	2–3	Talking (even singing) is easy.
Moderate	4–5	You can still chat but with more effort. You can feel your heart beating and your breathing is somewhat louder and faster.
Challenging	6–7	You can clearly hear yourself breathing; your heart is thumping and you're not inclined to chat.
Very challenging	8–9	You are panting, your heart is hammering, and conversation is nearly impossible.
Near maximum to maximum	10	You cannot sustain this effort for more than a few seconds.

As the chart illustrates, the *low intensity* we recommend doesn't allow for putting your feet up and grabbing the remote. An RPE of 5–6 means putting forth an effort that leaves you somewhat breathless and slightly sweaty but that still feels manageable (and equals 50–60 percent of your max heart rate). *High intensity* means pushing yourself to the point that you can barely speak, your heart is thumping in your chest, and you are soaked, if not dripping, with sweat. On a scale of 1–10, with 10 being the hardest you can work, you want to aim for an effort between 7 and 9 when you do the high-intensity intervals in this workout. (On the heart rate monitor, that's equal to 70–90 percent of your max heart rate.)

The Right Ratio

Nearly all of our workouts are based on some variation of interval training. The Cardio QUICK routine described in this chapter is an important part of your weight-loss program because it's pure cardio. Though the intensity varies, the movement is continuous so your heart rate stays elevated and you never stop burning calories. Plus, the low-intensity segments are a way to help your muscles flush out waste products, such as lactic acid, that build up during the high-intensity portions.

The intervals in this workout use 60-second patterns, where you devote 40 seconds to a moderate-intensity version of a movement and then hit it hard for 20 seconds with a high-intensity variation of the same movement. Each movement pattern is worked once, with no break in between (or as little as possible); then they are immediately run through again. This takes you to the 10-minute mark.

We've found this is the perfect blend of fast and slower movement for the majority of exercisers because you push your body to the limit for just the right amount of time before "resting" during the next moderate-intensity segment. This ensures you squeeze every last drop of calorie-burning goodness from 10 tiny minutes without going overboard.

If you aren't able to tolerate the high-intensity hits when you first try this workout, no worries. Simply do the moderate-intensity portion for the full 1 minute, take breaks as needed, or try the easier "Simplify It" suggestion for each movement pattern. Once you can tolerate this well, gradually start adding high-intensity portions, even if only for a few seconds to start. You'll be amazed how quickly your fitness improves and how soon you'll be glancing over the "Advance It" tips to make your workout even more challenging.

CARDIO QUICK WORKOUT

Keep in Mind
- follow the weekly recommendations for this workout based on the exercise level you chose in chapter 2
- repeat the circuit twice through with no rest in between; the warm-up is built into the first interval
- finish your final interval by walking in place for a few seconds to catch your breath if needed

What You Need
- nothing, unless you choose to use an interval timer (see "Time to Train" on page 45)

What to Expect
- to burn up to 110 calories with this workout

Interval 1 and 6

Jacks

Start: Stand with your feet together, elbows bent and in by your rib cage, palms facing forward so that your arms are opened into a W position.

40 seconds low intensity: Step your right foot out to the side, so your feet are slightly wider than hip width apart as you press and extend your arms overhead into a V shape, palms facing forward. Next, step your left foot into your right, bringing your feet and arms back into the start position. That's one rep. Alternate stepping right then left as quickly as you can for 40 seconds.

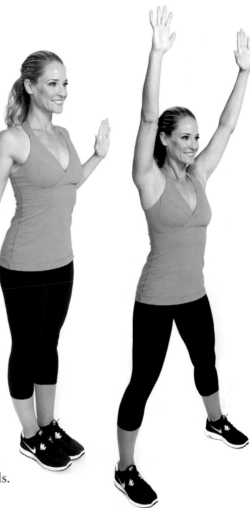

Set Time Chart

Interval 1: Jacks	1 minute
Interval 2: Skaters	1 minute
Interval 3: Up/Down	1 minute
Interval 4: Plank Ski	1 minute
Interval 5: Scissor Pickup	1 minute
Repeat Circuit:	5 minutes
TOTAL TIME	**10 MINUTES**

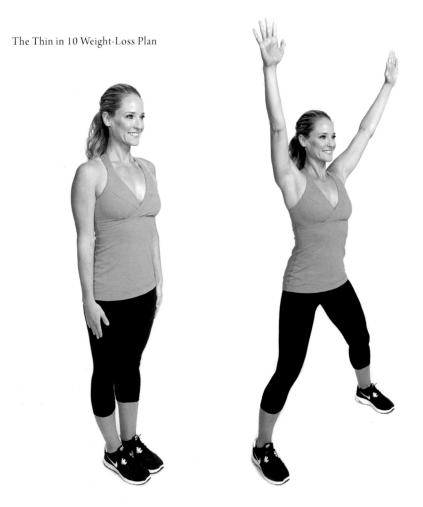

20 seconds high intensity: Jump your feet slightly wider than hip width apart as you raise your arms overhead, palms facing forward. Jump back to the start. Continue doing these jumping jacks for 20 seconds.

Ⓢimplify It:

Instead of jumping during the high-intensity interval, continue with the low-intensity jacks.

Ⓐdvance It:

Power up your jacks by bending your knees in the start position and then jumping up—opening legs wider than hip width apart in the air and making a wide circle with your arms in front of your body to help propel yourself off the ground. Land back in start position.

Interval 2 and 7
Skaters

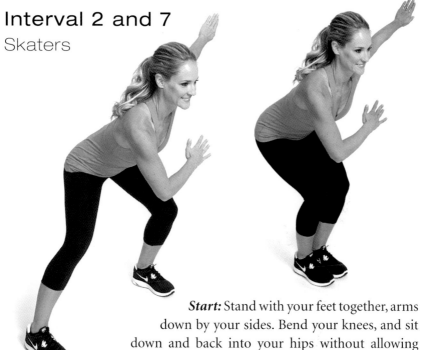

Start: Stand with your feet together, arms down by your sides. Bend your knees, and sit down and back into your hips without allowing your knees to move forward of your toes.

40 seconds low intensity: Keeping your body low and your knees bent, take a wide step to the right, sweeping both arms down and then to the right side (as if you were skating) from the front of your body out to the side, gliding your left foot into the right; then step to the left and reverse it. Repeat this as many times as you can for 40 seconds.

Time to Train

When timing your intervals, it can get rather clumsy to keep checking your watch. Jessica is in love with a little interval timer called the GYM-BOSS, which you can place nearby or clip to your clothing. This inexpensive, easy-to-use gadget can be programmed to beep at just about any repeating interval pattern (to learn more, visit www.thinin10.com). There are also a ton of smart phone and iPad interval timer apps that serve the same purpose. Basic apps that you can set for a single timing pattern are free. Those with the cool bells and whistles, including several developed by the same company that makes GYMBOSS, cost only a couple of bucks. It's definitely worth your time to check them out.

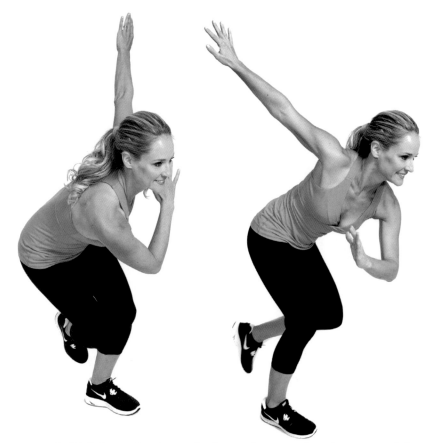

20 seconds high intensity: Instead of stepping your feet, leap your right foot out to the side as wide as you can, bringing your left foot behind your right leg, without tapping the floor. Keep your body low and knees bent, sweeping both arms across your body to the right as you leap. Then, push off with your right leg and leap to the left, reversing the arm sweep, as if you were skating. Do this as many times as you can for 20 seconds.

Ⓢimplify It:

Instead of adding the leap, speed up your side-to-side steps and make your arm motions larger.

Ⓐdvance It:

Make your leaps wider and faster.

Interval 3 and 8
Up/Down

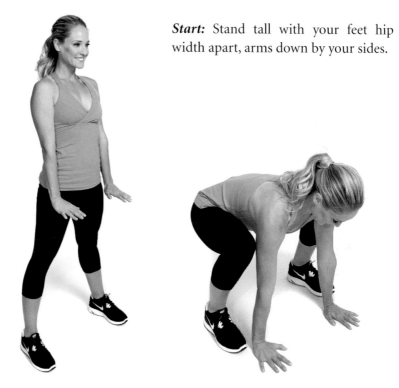

Start: Stand tall with your feet hip width apart, arms down by your sides.

40 seconds low intensity: Bend both of your knees, squat down, and, keeping your heels on the floor if you can, tap your hands to the floor. Quickly stand back up to start position. Repeat as many times as you can for 40 seconds.

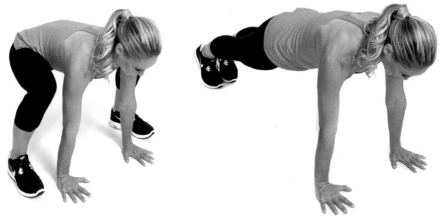

20 seconds high intensity: Lower to the floor and press your palms into the ground, keeping both arms straight and under your shoulders. Quickly step your right foot behind you and then your left, ending in the top of a push-up (or plank) position. Next, jump both feet back toward your hands, and then quickly stand back up to the start as you reach your arms straight overhead, palms facing forward. Repeat as many times as you can for 20 seconds.

Ⓢimplify It:

As you are coming out of your plank position, walk your feet in one at a time before standing up instead of jumping your feet back.

Ⓐdvance It:

Instead of walking both feet out to, the plank position, jump your feet back into the plank. When you stand up, add a small leap at the top, reaching both arms overhead and toward the ceiling as you jump.

Interval 4 and 9
Plank Ski

Start: Kneel on all fours with your palms directly beneath your shoulders and knees directly beneath your hips. Shift your weight into your arms, tighten your core, and straighten your legs so that you're in a plank position with your body forming a straight line from the top of your head to your heels.

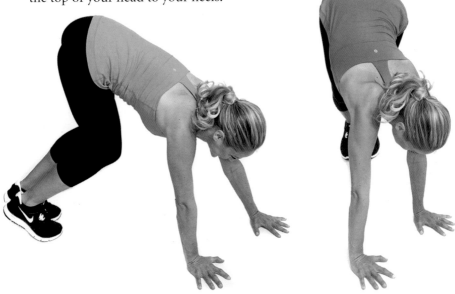

40 seconds low intensity: Bend both knees, shift your weight into your hands, and step your right foot and then your left a few feet to the right, moving into the 4 o'clock position, allowing your hips to rise into the air higher than your shoulders. Then quickly step your left foot and then your right over a few feet to the left into the 8 o'clock position. Repeat as many times as you can for 40 seconds.

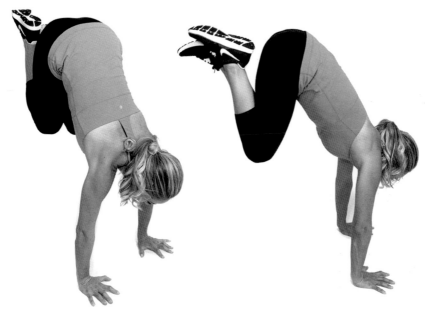

20 seconds high intensity: Instead of stepping your feet, jump both feet from side to side, landing lightly on the balls of your feet, keeping your shoulders over your hands, and pressing your hips into the air. Repeat as many times as you can for 20 seconds.

Ⓢimplify It:

Instead of jumping during the high-intensity portion, keep stepping feet side to side, increasing your speed.

Ⓐdvance It:

Make your jumps larger by kicking your heel toward your buttocks as you jump off the floor. Land lightly on the ball of your foot and then continue alternating "butt kicks" side to side.

Interval 5 and 10
Scissor Pickup

Start: Stand tall with your feet wider than hip width apart, your toes turned out about 45 degrees, and your arms down by your sides.

40 seconds low intensity: Sit into a squat as you reach down and forward so your right arm is in front of your legs and your left leg is behind them, tapping the ground with your right hand. Quickly stand back up and repeat, switching arms. Repeat as many times as you can, quickly, for 40 seconds.

20 seconds high intensity: Repeat the bend and reach with your right arm, but as you straighten your legs, jump your legs together, crossing your right leg in front of your left, landing on the balls of your feet. Quickly jump both feet back out to start position, bend your knees and lower yourself, reaching with your left arm this time, and repeat the scissor jump with your left leg crossing in front. Repeat this, alternating legs and arms each time, as many times as you can for 20 seconds.

Simplify It:

Instead of scissoring your legs during the high-intensity portion, simply jump your feet together and apart.

Advance It:

During the high-intensity portion, jump even higher before landing into the bent-knee position and then touching the floor.

Progress It

The beauty of sticking with an exercise routine is that you see results in so many forms—weight loss, better stamina, stronger muscles. When this workout ceases to challenge you, even when you're doing the most advanced versions of each move, tweak the intensity upward in these three ways:

1. ***Flip the interval times*** so that you're doing high intensity for 40 seconds and low intensity for 20 seconds. You can start by doing a 30:30 split to see how it goes.
2. ***Add a light hand weight*** (2–5 pounds) to the Jacks, Skaters, Up/Downs, and Scissor Pickups. You want to add just enough weight to feel the extra work but not so much it slows you down or throws off your form.
3. ***You'll lose weight*** even if you don't increase the amount of time you work out, but you may want to add an extra session here and there to move things along. Repeat the workout if you have the time. Or add it on a day when it's not scheduled.

Heart Math

If you find numbers motivating, monitoring your heart rate during exercise may inspire you to push yourself even harder. The most common way to determine your "target heart rate training zone" is with the heart rate max formula:

- Subtract your age from 220. That's your maximum heart rate.
- To estimate your target zone, multiply this number by a percentage: For example, if you're thirty years old and want to know what 60 percent of your maximum heart rate is, use this calculation:

$$220 - 30 = 190$$
$$190 \text{ x } .60 = 114 \text{ beats per minute}$$

This formula is easy, even if you aren't smarter than a fifth-grader in math, but it's not precise and can be off by as much as fifteen beats per minute. Other more complicated formulas exist but they, too, have proven to be of questionable accuracy.

If you plan on using a heart rate as an indicator of intensity—many serious fitness people do—get tested by a knowledgeable fitness or medical professional. Typically, this involves riding an exercise bike or walking on a treadmill as a sophisticated monitor measures your heart rate. The data gathered from this test reveals how fast your heart beats while you're in motion and provides you with your own personal training zone chart. You can then wear a heart monitor to help ensure you work out in your personal training zones.

Wrap-Up

Even after doing the Cardio QUICK workout for a while now, both of us find it energizing and inspiring. We hope it leaves you feeling the same way. If you're unable to complete the entire routine when you first try it, not to worry. Let the goal of conquering this routine fuel your ambition. And remember—you can swap this workout for the Cardio Quickie workout on the DVD and get the same great results.

CHAPTER

4 | # Simple
Strength

"Even though this is a short routine you can definitely tell you did a workout!"
—Keri, original *Thin in 10* focus group member

When you lose weight, not all of what you shed is fat. You lose muscle too. People who restrict their diets without exercising tend to lose the greatest amount of muscle.

The problem with this is that muscle is a more metabolically active tissue than fat. Although studies haven't been able to pinpoint an exact number, a pound of muscle burns about ten to thirty more calories per day than a pound of fat. This may sound miniscule, but it actually makes a vast difference in whether or not the scales tip in your favor.

If too much of your weight loss involves muscle mass, it is more difficult to keep on losing and inevitably your weight plateaus. Because your resting metabolism is now slower, maintaining the weight loss is also a struggle. Worse, if you gain pounds back, you may have a higher percentage of body fat the second time around, making your former weight more challenging to maintain! Yo-yo dieters fare the worst; the constant cycle of gaining and losing seems to grind down their resting metabolisms to a virtual halt.

Adding cardio exercise helps burn calories and can increase your metabolism for several hours following a workout, but it's not necessarily the best activity for preserving and building muscle. That's where your Simple Strength workouts come in.

Your Weight-Loss Secret Weapon

The only reliable way to keep your muscle at a steady percentage of your body weight is with strength training. Simple Strength is an introduction to strength training, even though it doesn't involve using any extra resistance like a dumbbell, barbell, or rubber tube to start. Even if you have been following another strength training routine, your body provides all the resistance you need to make the exercises challenging and is enough to help you build strength and muscle. As part of your *Thin in 10* body makeover, this simple strength workout helps preserve muscle so your metabolism continues to burn bright. If you give these workouts your all and do them consistently—as well as the other strength building workouts presented in this book—it's even possible to increase muscle mass as you lower body fat, which can result in a boost to your natural calorie burn.

Strength training helps transform your body in other ways too. Since muscle is denser than fat, it takes up less room—so more muscle translates to a firmer, tighter, and fitter body whether or not the needle on the scale budges. While it's impossible to selectively lose body fat from a particular area, strength training is the one activity that allows you to "spot train" a specific muscle group and thereby give it a smaller, tighter, firmer appearance. Strong muscles improve posture by providing the strength and support to help you stand up straighter—so you look thinner just by holding yourself up in a longer, leaner, more confident way. Have we convinced you of the powers of strength training yet?

Working It Out

"Anything worth doing is worth doing well." You've probably heard this wise old saying a thousand times, first from your mother, then your teachers, your boss . . . and now from us. Proper form is your best defense against injury and your biggest assurance that your workout delivers the results you came for. Performing each and every exercise correctly dramatically decreases the risk of hurting yourself and targets your muscles more effectively.

Each exercise comes with its own particular style pointers, but the ABCs of good exercise technique are based on common sense and a few fundamental rules. Always move through an exercise carefully; never lose control of your movement. Challenge yourself but don't go overboard. Avoid pushing yourself to do exercises that are beyond your ability and fitness level. And, of course, the golden rule of exercise: If it hurts, don't do it!

Your goal is to get through 1 minute of each exercise with good form. At the end of each set, you should feel worked but not completely spent. Aim for an intensity level somewhere between 7 and 8 on the RPE scale. For review on RPE, go to page 40. After you finish the set, repeat it with little to no rest if possible, to keep your heart rate elevated (translation: burn more calories). Do the exercises in the order they're listed; then move to the top of the rotation and repeat the entire sequence.

When the first version of an exercise becomes easy, you know what to do—move on! Try the next hardest version or look at the "Progress It" options for more ideas on challenging yourself. And, if you are advanced, feel free to start at level 4. Strength training gives you the best results when you give it your all. This may be only 10 minutes of working out, but it's a super-effective way to build strength and make fat vanish.

Long Is Wrong

"Long, lean muscles" and "strength without bulk" are promises advertised by some studios and trainers who teach yoga, Pilates, or dance. These claims imply strength training bulks you up. Don't be fooled! You are born with a certain body type and no matter how much or what kind of exercise you do, your muscles will develop within their natural length and shape. It's impossible to change the length of your muscles. That myth was probably started (and is still perpetuated) by instructors who are naturally predisposed to willowy physiques. They may have the mistaken impression that this is the result of their training and don't realize it won't materialize for many of their clients. You can make significant and magnificent improvements to your body with all types of exercise, no matter what your natural body type is.

SIMPLE STRENGTH WORKOUT

Keep in Mind
- follow the weekly recommendations for this workout based on the exercise level you chose in chapter 2

What You Need
- nothing, unless you prefer to use a mat or towel to lie down on for the floor exercises

What to Expect
- to burn up to ninety calories with this workout

Set Time Chart

W & V Squats	1 minute
Cross Tap Push-Ups	1 minute
Extend & Row	1 minute
Figure-8 Lunges	1 minute
Plank & Tuck	1 minute
Repeat Circuit	5 minutes
TOTAL TIME	**10 MINUTES**

If you're able, repeat the circuit twice through with no break in between. The warm-up and cool-down are built into the movements. You can gradually build your range of motion.

Interval 1 and 6
W & V Squats

Start: Stand with your feet together and your elbows bent and held to your sides so that your arms are slightly open in a W position with palms facing your body.

Move: Step your right foot out to the side, so that your feet are hip width apart, and then bend your knees and sit back into your hips to lower your body (as if you're about to sit in a chair). As you lower yourself, reach your arms overhead into a V shape, with your arms extended on either side of your ears and your palms facing in. Keep your core strong and your body-weight evenly distributed between your toes and heels. Lower as far down as you can without letting your knees push past your toes, and keep your chin in toward your chest (to avoid straining your neck). Once you've reached your lowest point, press through your feet and stand back up to the start,

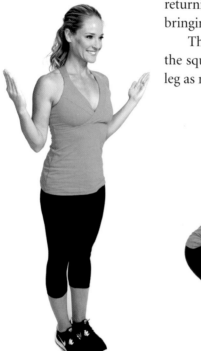

returning your arms to the W position and bringing your feet back together.

That's one rep. Alternate stepping into the squat with your right and then your left leg as many times as you can for 1 minute.

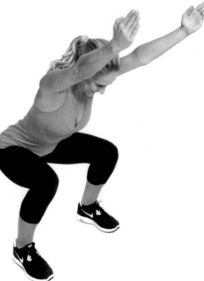

Simplify It:

Instead of stepping into the squat, keep your feet stationary and hip width apart as you squat.

Advance It:

Add power to this move. As you rise out of your squat, push off the floor with both feet and jump back into the start position; then lift both feet off the floor at once, and quickly land in a squat position on the other side. Keep your arm movements the same as above.

Interval 2 and 7
Cross Tap Push-Ups

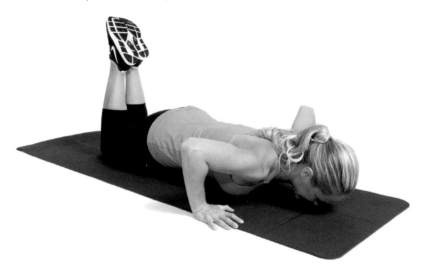

Start: Kneel on the floor with your palms slightly forward and to the sides of your shoulders and knees directly beneath your hips. Keeping your spine straight and chin tucked toward your chest, lift your lower legs off the floor (so that just your knees lightly touch the ground) and point your toes. Now, shift your weight forward onto your hands until most, but not all, of your weight is on your hands and the rest of your weight is supported by your thighs just above your knees. (You may need to walk your hands forward to achieve the right balance.)

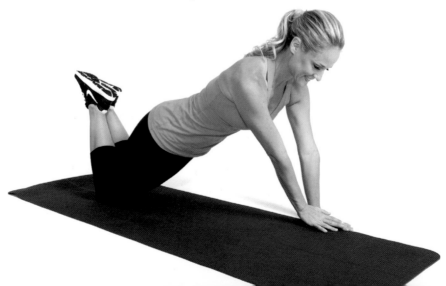

Move: While maintaining a straight spine and strong core, bend your elbows out to the side and lower your chest to the floor. Tap your chest lightly on the floor, and then press back up. As you press up and away from the floor, bring your left hand over and tap the back of your right palm. Quickly return your left hand to your start position and immediately start another push-up.

That's one rep. Alternate your tapping hand after each push-up, as many times as you can for 1 minute.

Ⓢimplify It:

Do your push-ups from an all-fours kneeling position.

Ⓐdvance It:

Do your push-ups on your toes, with legs fully extended in a full plank position.

Interval 3 and 8
Extend & Row

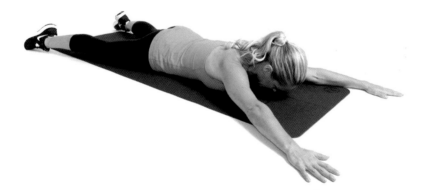

Start: Lie facedown on the floor, with your arms and legs spread out to form an X shape, palms and toes resting on the floor.
Move: While maintaining a strong core, lift your arms, chest, and legs off the floor into a hovering "skydive" position. Keep your chin tucked toward your chest, eyes looking down at the floor. Now, with your chest and thighs still lifted, "row" your arms by bending your elbows and pulling your arms

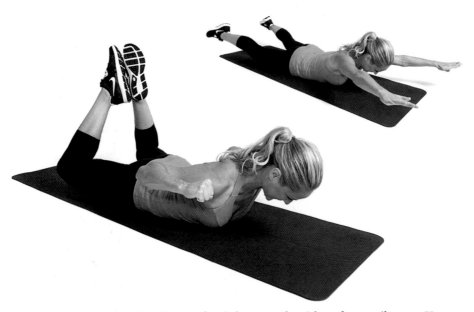

(tightening your hands into fists) down to the sides of your rib cage. Keeping your thighs off the floor and your toes pointed, simultaneously bend your knees and curl your heels into your body. Stretch your arms and legs back out to the skydive position (allow your hands to open, with palms facing the ground, as your arms extend) and then lower your chest and thighs back to the starting X position.

That's one rep. Do as many repetitions as you can, with good form, for 1 minute.

Ⓢimplify It:

Let your thighs rest on the floor and focus on lifting just your arms and chest off the floor to perform the arm row.

Ⓐdvance It:

Instead of lowering yourself to the ground after each row, stay in the lifted skydive position and continue reps for 1 minute.

Interval 4 and 9
Figure-8 Lunges

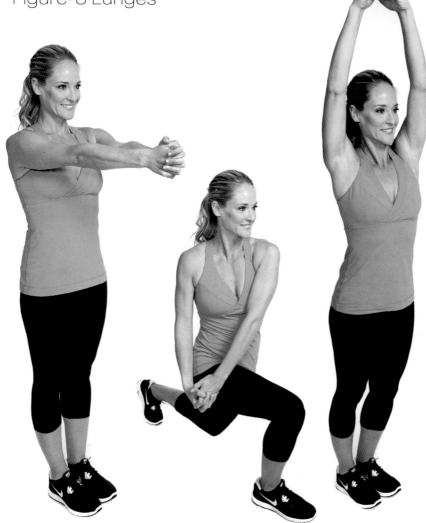

Start: Stand with your feet together, core tight, with your arms straight out in front of your chest, hands clasped together.

Move: Keeping your back straight and eyes looking straight ahead, step your right leg a stride's length forward into a lunge position, bending both knees about 90 degrees and then step back to the start position. As you step forward, reach your arms to the right across your body and "scoop" them down toward the outside of your right hip. As you step back to start, complete the figure-eight movement with your arms by scooping them up and back in front of your chest. Repeat to the left side.

That's one rep. Do as many repetitions as you can, with good form, for 1 minute.

(S)implify It:

Instead of making a figure-eight motion with your arms, simply keep them extended straight out in front of you (in the start position) as you alternate lunges.

(A)dvance It:

Instead of stepping into your lunges, add a switch lunge jump while continuing your figure-eight arm movement: Push off with your right leg as you rise out of the lunge, jump both feet off the ground, and quickly switch legs, landing in a lunge position with your left leg in front. Your arms should cross over your body and "scoop" as you land.

The *Thin in Ten* Advantage: Beyond Beauty

This Simple Strength workout does good things for your body far beyond firming your thighs and tightening your buns: It's heart healthy too! Cardio exercise is necessary for increasing the stamina and efficiency of heart muscles, but it's strength training that makes them stronger. Strength training generates a lot of force in your muscles, the heart muscles included. This extra force creates "micro tears" in the cardiac fiber. When the tears repair, the fibers grow back more powerful than before so your heart is able to pump blood more forcefully.

The benefits don't stop there either. Science is finding that strength training can lift depression, raise good cholesterol, and improve cognitive function.[10] It's been shown to fight diabetes by elevating the protein that clears glucose from the blood and transports it into the skeletal muscle, giving the muscles more energy and lowering overall blood sugar levels. Fierce, focused workouts like a 10-minute Simple Strength session deliver every health advantage that strength training has to offer.

Interval 5 and 10
Plank & Tuck

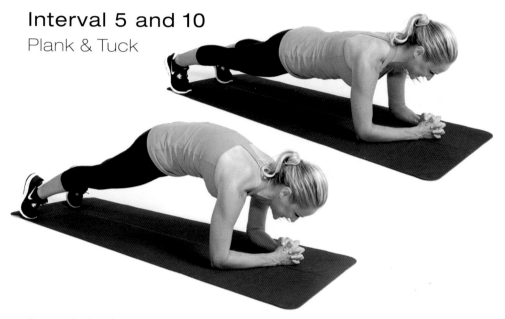

Start: Lie facedown on the floor, with your arms bent, elbows aligned beneath your shoulders, and hands clasped together. Lift your chest off the floor by propping yourself up on your forearms. Tuck your toes under, tighten your core, and lift your hips and thighs off the floor so your spine forms a straight line from the top of your head to your heels.

Move: Press your shoulders down, and tilt your pelvis under (imagine scooping your belly button into your back). As you tuck your pelvis, focus on using your abdominals, not your glutes, to tuck under and shift your weight forward into your arms and into your toes, allowing your heels to lift a little higher and your butt up to lift higher toward the ceiling. Hold this position for one count and then shift your weight back slightly to your starting full plank position.

That's one rep. Repeat as many times as you can for 1 minute.

Simplify It:

Keep your knees bent and lightly touching the ground for more support in your plank position.

Advance It:

Alternate lifting one leg slightly off the floor at the top of the movement.

Progress It

Lifting your own body weight is plenty challenging, especially when you are new to strength training. And make no mistake, it provides enough resistance to produce the results you want. Depending on how you move or angle yourself, you can make an exercise harder without adding any additional resistance. Still, when a strength exercise becomes effortless, it's time to progress it. That's the only way to keep on seeing improvements. If you're at that point, try one of these three strategies:

1. *Pick up a weight.* Adding some resistance to the moves in the form of a dumbbell definitely gets your muscles' attention. Use a weight that's heavy enough so you feel worked by the end of a set, but not so heavy that you can't maintain your form. For most people, that's between three and eight pounds depending on the exercise. (Note that resistance is also included in the Total Body Circuit coming up in chapter 5.)

2. *Lose the rest.* Move from one exercise to the next with no break in between. Doing this gives the workout a cardio element, so besides pushing your muscles, you pump up calorie burn as well.

3. *Slow it down.* If you like depending on just your body to do the work, slow down the portion of the exercise where you exert the most effort. For instance, lower yourself extra slowly when you do W & V Squats. You may do fewer reps but feel the exercise even more. You can combine this strategy with weights or bands too.

Hurts So Good

Muscle soreness is the "good pain" you feel when you've pressed your muscles past the point they normally work, causing tiny tears and swelling within the muscle fibers. It's often referred to as delayed onset muscle soreness, or DOMS, because the dull ache that spreads out across the muscle usually peaks one or two days after a particularly hard workout. Some residual stiffness can remain for up to a week. Typical remedies are ice, hot showers, stretching, pain relievers such as aspirin, and massage.

Hurts So Good   continued

But the healing powers of time seem to be the only reliable way to find complete relief.

While an occasional bout of DOMS means your workouts continue to challenge, you shouldn't experience it so frequently that it interferes with your life or so severely that you can't comb your hair or walk down a flight of stairs without wincing. If that's what's happening, consider backing off or taking a few days' rest. If the muscle pain you feel is sharp and pinpointed, assume it's the result of an injury to a muscle, tendon, or ligament and see a doctor.

Wrap-Up

It's great to feel strong. Sure you look better—your body is tighter, firmer, and smaller. But nothing beats the empowerment of lifting, pushing, and pulling things in your everyday life in ways you never thought possible. For example, that heavy door to your office building that you've always struggled to open? After doing this program for a while, you may feel like you can rip it off its hinges. And that's just one example of the type of improvements that are possible. It's amazing what you can accomplish in a mere 10 minutes, isn't it? Oh, and for a terrific alternative to this work-out, try the DVD Strength Shot workout.

CHAPTER

5

The 10-Minute
Total Body Circuit

"If you're pressed for time, this workout is perfect!
It's 10 minutes and you can get on with your life."
—Sarah, original *Thin in 10* focus group member

Strength training is important for preserving muscle. Total Body Circuit builds on what you learned about strength training in chapter 4, but this type of exercise involves moving at a faster pace and using additional resistance. Speedy exercise used to be considered a bad thing, like driving too fast or gulping down a meal. That philosophy has changed. Research now shows that spending some time in the fitness fast lane while keeping good form improves results.

Circuit training is a perfect example of how velocity can work in your favor. It is like a cross between a kick-butt strength workout and a take-no-prisoners cardio routine. Total Body Circuit keeps you moving the entire time at a cardio pace. Each set of reps is slow and controlled, but in between sets, you move at a lightning pace, switching from one exercise to the next with no break. The emphasis is on both hustle *and* muscle.

Calorie-Burning Blitz

When done at a manageable but rapid pace, strength training turbocharges calorie burn during the workout. Total Body Circuit annihilates calories, especially when compared to conventional weight training, where you take your time and rest between sets to fully recover. Conventional training burns a respectable forty to sixty calories in 10 minutes, but studies done on behalf of the American Council on Exercise show you can burn nearly one hundred calories with the same time spent doing high-intensity circuit training.[11] That figure rivals the burn you get from high-octane cardio activities such as running, power walking, and doing our pure cardio workout.

"Dieters who don't take steps to preserve muscle mass often hit a plateau."

Metabolism is key when discussing calorie burning, weight loss, and weight training. *Metabolism* is one of those words like SPF (sun protection factor) or antioxidants: Some of us use it in conversation, as in "I wish I had a faster metabolism," but are not quite sure what the term means. The simple definition of metabolism is the rate at which the body burns calories. Its largest component is known as resting metabolism; about 70 percent of the total calories you burn daily are used to pump blood, regenerate cells, and power all the other automatic body functions that keep you alive. The rest of your calorie burn is largely devoted to activities such as digestion and movement.

Strength training influences your resting metabolism. How so? It packs on muscle, which helps offset the muscle loss that inevitably occurs when you lose weight. When it comes to weight loss, muscle is important because it burns slightly more calories per pound than fat. Dieters who don't take steps to preserve muscle mass often hit a plateau—they stop losing weight, even if they're doing a good job of limiting calories. Worse, some find they can't even maintain the weight they have lost while eating fewer calories.

Studies show that when weight training is high energy, like the workout in this chapter, its benefits go beyond burning a certain number of calories during a workout by further elevating metabolism after you've finished working out—and this metabolism boost can last for several hours to several days. This can result in an additional fifteen to three hundred calories burned long after you've hit the showers. Just how many extra calories you shed as a result of this metabolic "after burn" effect isn't clear. Different studies have produced very different results. But even if the after burn is at the low end, we'll take it. At the very least, it seems to translate to a 15 percent calorie burn bonus without additional effort. Maybe that's more like buying two cans of veggies at the supermarket and getting the third for free than winning a car—but still. Every little bit helps when you're trying to lose weight and reshape your body. The proof is mounting that small metabolic shifts can help make a significant difference in your weight-loss efforts.

Serious Sculpt and Stamina

The circuit routine described in this chapter asks you to take little or no rest between sets of exercises so you hit every major muscle group in 10 minutes. Remember, a repetition is one complete movement of an exercise and a set is a group of repetitions. Move quickly between sets and do each repetition within a set slowly, carefully, and with good form. The resistance you use is relatively light at first, but the lack of rest between sets increases the intensity—so you build total body strength and sharpen the shape and firmness of your muscles as though you worked with significantly heavier weights and did fewer repetitions.

This type of workout comes with some pretty awesome cardio benefits too. Circuit training rockets you into the sweat zone right from the start. Your heart pumps and your lungs expand the same way they do during a cardio session. In fact, circuit training elicits and sustains heart rates and oxygen usage, just like running, cycling, and other traditional cardio activities, and it does a great job of whipping you into aerobic shape. The American College of Sports Medicine gives circuit training a thumbs-up for increasing endurance and improving cardiorespiratory health.[12]

Ready, Set, Go

Now that we've convinced you that circuit training rocks, let's cover some of the basics so you can try it for yourself. For the 10-Minute Total Body Circuit workout you need the following:

- a band, tube, or substitute (see pages 76 and 81)
- a clock, stopwatch, or wristwatch with a timer

If you can set your timing device to beep every minute, do so. It's easier to keep moving and concentrate on what you're doing if you don't have to keep eyeballing the time.

That brings us to the next point. As with all of the *Thin in 10* workouts, rather than counting reps, time each set instead. Each set lasts for 1 minute. If you choose, you can work both sides of your body on each interval for a total of 2 minutes. (See the Set Time Chart at the beginning of the workout, on page 71.) When the time allotted for a set is up, move right into the next exercise. If you must catch your breath, try to take no more than a 15-second break.

However, if you're new to exercise, particularly high-intensity exercise like this routine, it's okay to rest longer if you need it. The goal isn't to make you pass out; it's to push yourself up to but not over the edge of your comfort zone, to elevate your heart rate, and to give your muscles a run for their money. If you don't need a break, you should go for it. Eventually, you'll be able to jump seamlessly from set to set with no rest at all, doing the most challenging version of each move. When you can do that, not to worry—we've got plenty of other ways to challenge you. Aim for an intensity level between 7 and 9 on the RPE chart. (For a refresher on RPE, see page 40.)

> "Aim for an intensity level between 7 and 9 on the RPE chart."

Each move included in this workout engages multiple muscle groups at once. We designed it this way so you get the most effective and efficient total body workout possible. Also, every move involves the lower body because most of your metabolism-boosting muscle mass is located in your butt, hips, and thighs. The extra emphasis on this area ensures faster lower-body toning results and, actually, faster results overall. We can all get on board with that!

On your Total Body Circuit days, be sure to do the routine twice through—once in the morning and once in the afternoon or evening. This creates a slight caloric advantage by giving you two shots of metabolic after burn rather than just one.

Oh, one more very important point before you hit this circuit: Keep your movements controlled. Aim to move quickly from one set to the next but don't race through the individual repetitions. Perform your movements carefully and through a full range of motion, the same as you would during any strength training routine. Never toss technique and safety by the wayside. Control each rep, use impeccable form, but keep up your overall pace.

THE 10-MINUTE TOTAL BODY CIRCUIT

Keep in Mind
- follow the weekly recommendations for this workout based on the exercise level you chose in chapter 2

What You Need
- a resistance band (you can substitute dumbbells or other weighted objects such as water bottles)

What to Expect
- to burn up to 100 calories with this workout
- to build or maintain muscle mass

Set Time Chart

Warm-Up	30 seconds
Pickup Press	1 minute
Bow & Fly	2 minutes
Scoop & Push	2 minutes
Down & X	2 minutes
Press & Tap	1 minute
Reach & Lift	1 minute
Cool-Down	30 seconds
TOTAL TIME	**10 MINUTES**

Warm-Up
Knee Lift with Arm Circles
(30 seconds)

Start: Stand with your feet hip width apart and arms down by your sides. Lift your right knee toward your chest as you reach your slightly bent arms forward and up, making large circles in the air with them. Alternate knees, making one circle per knee lift.

Interval 1
Pickup Press
(1 minute)

Start: Hold one end (or handle) of your band in each hand and stand tall on the center of the band with your feet hip width apart, so there is an even amount of band on either side. Bend your elbows and lift your bent arms so your elbows are level with your rib cage and palms are facing in toward your body.

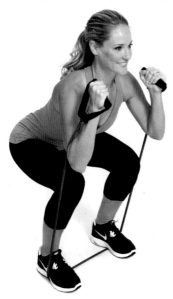

Move: Sit back into your hips (as if you're about to sit into a chair) as you bend your knees, lowering your body. Keep your abs drawn in and keep your body weight evenly distributed between your toes and heels. Lower your body as far as you can without letting your knees push past your toes. Once you've reached your lowest point, press through your feet and stand back up to the starting position, straightening your arms overhead and pressing the band toward the ceiling.

That's one rep. Be careful not to lock your knees or elbows at the end of your range of motion. Do as many reps as you can until the minute is up.

Simplify It:

Instead of standing with both feet on the band, lighten the resistance by placing only one foot on the center of the band.

Advance It:

For an additional core challenge, rotate from the waist to the right as you press overhead, return to center, and then rotate from the waist to the left on the next rep.

Progress It

You know it's time to make an exercise more challenging when you can do the maximum number of recommended repetitions with little effort. When you're at this point, don't rest on your laurels. It's important to push yourself so you continue to see improvements. To increase your intensity, you've got three choices:

1. *Switch to a more strenuous version of the exercise.* Look for the "Advance It" option.
2. *Tighten the band.* To do this, grip lower down on your band or otherwise shorten it to make it less stretchy and thus more difficult to pull taut. You can mark the band with a pen to keep track of where you typically grip it for each exercise.
3. *Switch to a band with greater resistance.* Generally, bands are color coded, with the darker bands offering the heaviest resistance.

Interval 2
Bow & Fly
(2 minutes)

Start: Stand tall with the center of the band placed securely under the arch of your left foot. Cross the ends, making an X with the band, and then grasp an end in each hand so there is an even amount of band on each side. With both legs straight, step your right leg about a stride's length behind you so your legs are in a "split stance." Shift your weight onto your front leg, bending your knees slightly, and lift your back heel off the floor. Hold your arms slightly in front of you, palms facing in.

Move: Keeping your back straight and abdominals tight, bend (or bow) forward until your chest is parallel to the floor. As you are bowing, open your arms to the sides and up to shoulder level, keeping your palms facing the floor. Bring your arms back in and straighten up to the start position, being sure to keep your back straight and your abdominals tight as you lift back up.

That's one rep. Repeat as many times as you can for 1 minute and then switch legs and repeat for 1 minute.

Ⓢimplify It:

Instead of stepping one leg behind you, keep your feet closer together for more stability.

Ⓐdvance It:

Add another core and balance challenge by lifting your back foot off the floor when bending forward.

Interval 3
Scoop & Push
(2 minutes)

Start: Hold an end of the band in each hand with your arms at your sides, elbows slightly bent, and palms facing forward. Stand tall with the band looped under the arch of your left foot, with an equal amount of band on either side.

Move: Step your right foot about a stride's length forward and bend your right knee. As you step, scoop your arms up in front of you to shoulder level, palms up. (Picture yourself holding a basket of clothes.)

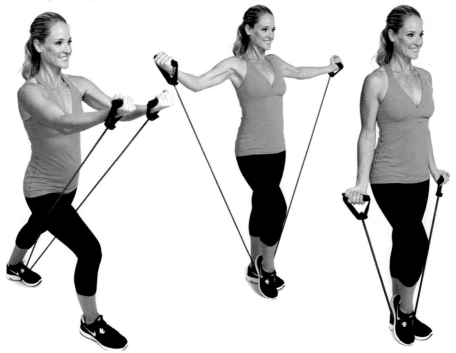

Draw your abdominals in, push off your right foot, and step it back beside your left foot. As you do this, open your arms to the sides. Maintain your arms at shoulder height, keeping the scoop shape of your arms as you move. Next, move both your arms and legs back to the start position.

That's one rep. Repeat for 1 minute with the band under your left foot and then switch and do 1 minute with the band under your right foot.

Ⓢimplify It:

Keep your feet stationary and perform only the arm movement.

Ⓐdvance It:

Instead of stepping your foot back, lift your right knee to hip height as you open your arms to the side. This challenges your core muscles and balance.

Band and Tube Buying Basics

Deluxe rubber resistance kits—complete with a variety of tubes, bands, handles, and attachments—may run a few hundred dollars, but you certainly don't need to get that fancy. A single band typically costs just a few dollars and is one of the least expensive and most easily stored pieces of resistance training equipment around. Several different types of bands are available. Some are made of flat pieces of rubber; others are tube shaped with handles on either end. They all can vary in resistance and thickness. Look for resistance levels between light and medium; we don't recommend using a heavy-duty band for this particular routine. For a better grip, you may want a tube with handles.

You can purchase exercise bands and tubes almost anywhere—at most sporting goods stores, big box stores, health food stores, and booksellers. Or you can shop for them on the following websites:

www.sprifitness.com
www.fitnesslifeline.com
www.performbetter.com
www.ripcords.com
www.bodylastics.com
www.gaiam.com

Interval 4

Down & X

(2 minutes)

Start: Stand tall and place the center of the band securely under the arch of your left foot, with an even amount of band on each side. Cross the ends of the band to make an X, and then grasp an end in each hand. Straighten your arms along your sides, palms facing.

Move: Lunge your right leg back about a stride's length and bend both knees so your left thigh is parallel to the floor and your left knee is perpendicular to it; be sure to keep your left knee tracking directly over your shoelace and your back heel lifted off the floor.

Next, hinge forward from your hips and shift your weight onto your left leg, keeping your back straight as your hands reach down to your front foot. Bring your body up, keeping your spine straight and abdominals tight, and raise your arms forward and up so the X shape of the band stretches taller and tauter. Be sure your palms are facing forward. Lunge back down and reach both hands to your front foot again.

That's one rep. Repeat for 1 minute and then switch legs and go for 1 more minute.

Simplify It:

Don't lunge as deeply and keep your feet stationary (don't shift forward but lift your heel as you perform the arm movement).

Advance It:

Lunge deeper and lift your back foot completely off the floor as your arms make the X shape.

Interval 5
Press & Tap
(1 minute)

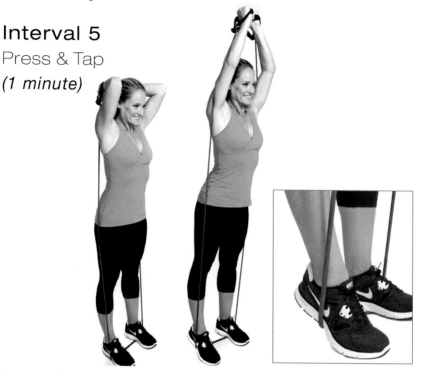

Start: Hold an end of the band in each hand and stand tall on the center of the band with your feet hip width apart; there should be an even amount of band on either side. Stretch your arms overhead and then bend your elbows to bring your hands behind your head and the band in back of you. Clasp the fingers of both hands together for more stability.

Move: Straighten your arms overhead to tighten the band and, as you do, shift your weight onto your right foot and lift your left heel off the floor. Bend your elbows again and lower your heel. Repeat, this time lifting your right heel off the floor.

That's one rep. Repeat as many times as you can for 1 minute, alternating legs.

Ⓢimplify It:

Skip the heel lift.

Ⓐdvance It:

Lift your entire foot off the floor and lift your leg a few inches up and out to the side.

Interval 6
Reach & Lift
(1 minute)

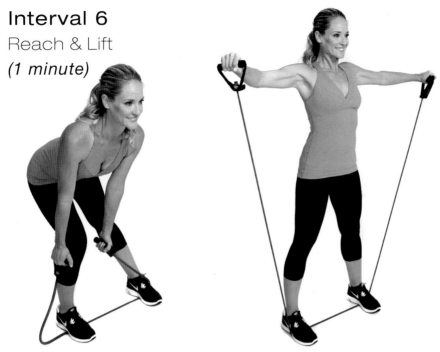

Start: Hold an end of the band in each hand and stand tall with both feet on the band in a wider-than-hip-width stance and an equal amount of band on each side. Relax your arms at your sides, palms facing.

Move: Shift into a side lunge to the right by bending your right knee and pushing your hips behind you, arms reaching down on either side of your knee.

Next, straighten your right knee and stand back up as you raise your arms up and out to the sides to shoulder level. Lower your arms as you shift into a left lunge and repeat.

That's one rep. Repeat as many times as you can for 1 minute, alternating sides.

Simplify It:

Alternate single arm shoulder raises and don't go as deep on your lunges.

Advance It:

Lunge and reach your hands to the floor, one on either side of your foot.

Totally Tubular

Exercise tubes and bands—made of strong, stretchy rubberized material—are super effective during workouts, especially when you use them properly. Follow these six tips to get the most from your rubber resistance—and your 10-Minute Total Body Circuit.

1. *Find the right resistance band.* While a heavier band may have worked well for you in the past, it may not be appropriate for the Total Body Circuit workout due to the large range of motion required for some of the moves. Remember, you don't have to buy a new band or tube; you can use the alternative moves if you have a band that is too heavy or none at all.

2. *Do each exercise slowly.* Even though you move quickly between exercises with as little rest as possible, you actually take your time as you lift and lower. Take the movement through the full range of motion. Not only is this safer but it's more effective because your muscles get the maximum workout possible.

3. *Hold on loosely.* When you hold the band or tube in your hand, don't wrap it so tightly around your palm that it's uncomfortable or cuts off your circulation. Wrap it loosely several times so there's a little space between your hand and the rubber but your grip is still secure.

4. *Press down firmly.* When you place the band or tube under your feet, be sure to step down firmly with the band beneath your instep. Trust us—you don't want it sliding out of place and snapping you in the crotch!

5. *Be safe.* Although you may substitute other items in place of a band, only use bands that are designed for exercising and don't use them for anything else but exercising.

6. *Take care of your equipment.* Inspect your band or tube frequently for holes and tears and replace it when it's reached the end of its life span. Store your band in a place that isn't too hot or too cold. Extreme temperatures may shorten the life of the rubber. Place it somewhere you'll see it often so it isn't forgotten or gathering dust.

Cool-Down
Alternating Waist Twists
(30 seconds)

Stand with your feet hip width apart, your arms extended in front of you at shoulder height, palms facing. Keeping your hips squared to the front, open your right arm and reach behind you as you twist your torso and look back over your right shoulder. Slowly return to the front and repeat to the left. Alternate sides for 30 seconds.

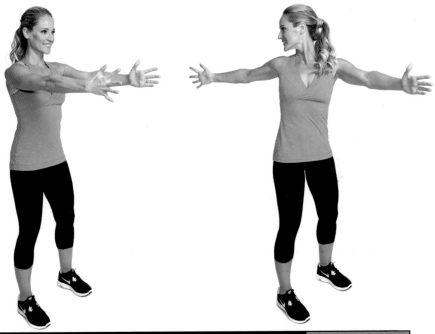

No Band? No Problem!

Don't sweat it if you don't have a band or tube. Or actually do sweat it—by using another form of resistance such as a dumbbell, weighted exercise ball, or any other weighted object you can hold safely and comfortably. If there's absolutely nothing handy to hold on to, don't let that stop you. You can switch to a more challenging version of each move or add an extra circuit to the routine. Besides, you may want to skip using resistance in the beginning until you learn the routine and build up some fitness.

The *Thin in 10* Advantage:
Nixing the "I Burned It, I Earned It" Syndrome

One 2009 study by a consortium of universities found that over-weight women volunteers lost about the same amount of weight whether they sat on their duffs all day or worked their tails off in the gym for more than three and a half hours a week.[13] Exercisers lost weight no faster than sloths because they ate more to compensate for their additional activity. Either they were truly hungrier upon exiting the gym or, psychologically, they felt they had earned the right to eat more after working up a sweat.

Scientists have long suspected that this "burn and earn" mentality is why even dedicated exercisers sometimes have trouble shedding pounds. Because all *Thin in 10* workouts take just 10 minutes, they are likely to help you avoid this problem. And while our workout plan is just as effective at revving your metabolism and burning overall calories as a much longer workout, 10-minute spurts won't stimulate hunger hormones and certainly won't lull you into that false sense of entitlement that makes you reach for an extra slice of pizza.

Wrap-Up

The Total Body Circuit workout was one of our testers' favorites. They also loved the Total Body Band DVD workout, which you can use as an alternative to this workout. They loved how it got their heart pounding and their muscles cranking. We're sure you'll feel the same. And just think—all it takes is a few ounces of rubber and 10 tiny minutes.

CHAPTER

6 | Core
& More

"I've definitely noticed my core is tighter since doing this workout"
—Sarah, original *Thin in 10* focus group member

Sculpted abs are like the coveted fashion accessory few people have but everyone wants. That's why we've included a special core workout as part of your *Thin in 10* program. We also know that anyone can improve the appearance of their midsection without spending hours and hours on a grueling workout routine. You need only 10 quick minutes to reshape your middle to its full potential. Here's why:

Many traditional ab workouts ask you to devote yourself to doing hundreds or even thousands of reps of isolation exercises such as the basic crunch. Researchers from San Diego State University who studied the best way to sculpt core muscles found that doing shorter, more intense routines is actually more effective, especially when you choose moves that really laser in on your midline.[14]

The exercises they rated tops use the larger abdominal and lower back muscles in combination with the smaller, deeper core muscles involved in stabilizing and rotating the trunk and work several middle muscle groups at once. We designed our Core & More routine to meet the San Diego State team's standards. This routine takes a less-is-more-effective approach to whittling away your middle. Our initial *Thin in 10* testers loved it!

The Secret (and Reality) of Fab Abs

Yes, everyone can improve the appearance of their belly—and in some cases achieve that coveted flatness—but we'd be lying if we didn't tell you that it takes hard work and dedication to make it happen. The 10-minute routine in this chapter is super-effective but core exercises alone won't be enough to achieve the abs of your dreams. Toning your middle involves lifestyle choices too.

> "Toning your middle involves lifestyle choices too."

Lowering your body fat is a big part of the equation. While the right exercises certainly help anchor the core muscles to the spine, the definition won't be visible if your middle is covered in excess fat. You need to burn off calories with the other workouts in this book, and you need to eat a healthy diet. It's easier if you follow our *Thin in 10* eating plan. For better or worse, Mother Nature has predisposed you to lose weight in a certain way and in a certain order. Even if you lose a substantial amount of weight, there's no telling how much of it will peel off the middle. Genetic tendencies, hormones, pregnancy, posture, and age factor into how easily you slim your waistline. However, that's not to say you can't work with, rather than against, your genetics. You may never be able to bounce grapes off a midsection that looks like it's been chiseled from stone, but a dedicated approach to this workout helps tighten and tone your middle to enviable proportions.

Core, Defined

For the record, your core is not the same as your abdominal muscles (abs). Core refers to the four layers of the abs (rectus abdominis, external and internal obliques, and transverse abdominis), hip flexors, spine extensors, hip adductors (inner thigh muscles), hip abductors (including gluteus medius), and multifidus. This is the entire collection of muscles that wrap around your torso. They allow you to twist, bend, and arch—and perhaps most important—they're responsible for stabilizing and supporting the entire spine. Ab muscles may be the showpiece in the group, but you've got to firm and strengthen all the core muscles if you want results worthy of crop tops.

Because your core is three dimensional, the basic crunch shouldn't be the main exercise in your core routine, even though it's been a longtime workout staple. In the first place, most of us spend a good part of the day hunched over a computer or steering wheel, so the spine is already in the constantly flexed position that can lead to poor posture and a weak core. Doing an excess of spine-flexing crunches only makes matters worse. Second, a straightforward crunch activates a very tiny part of the rectus abdominus, the long flat sheet of muscle that runs the length of your torso, from breastbone to hip. Devoting too much of what little workout time you have to such a miniscule patch of muscle is pointless. Also, as tests like those run by San Diego State show, there are many, many other exercises that do a superior job of toning core muscles.

Nonetheless, we think having a few crunch variations in a core routine is helpful. They're familiar, are easy to do, and require no special equipment. Plus, most people feel just about everything when they first begin working their middles; crunches are no exception. For these reasons, we've included one crunch-style exercise near the beginning of our Core & More routine as a way to warm up the rectus and prepare the core for the rest of the workout.

The Rules of Engagement

This Core & More routine includes ten killer core moves. Focus on quality rather than quantity to make every rep count. Remember, slower reps are almost always more effective for reaching the deepest muscle fibers; slapping through your reps as quickly possible just to be done gets you nowhere. If you can't do a full minute of a particular move with good form, take a break and start again when you have enough strength to do it right. A single rep done perfectly is worth a thousand reps done with sloppy technique.

When you're able to complete a full minute of an exercise effortlessly and with good form, congratulate yourself and then move on. Always push yourself to go to the next level as soon as you can. To help you with this, we've listed a more advanced version of each exercise.

During each repetition of each exercise, imagine you are trying to zip up a pair of skinny jeans that are three sizes too small—your core should feel braced, strong, and pulled inward throughout. To achieve this, tighten your tummy into your spine—especially that "cummerbund" region below the belly button—and hold it there for the entire set. Maintaining this firm core keeps your lower back from either sagging or arching. Be sure not to "cheat" the moves by pushing with your legs and tilting your pelvis upward. For best results, keep your pelvis parallel to the floor during most moves.

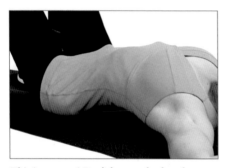

This is a no-no! Don't let your back arch or sag.

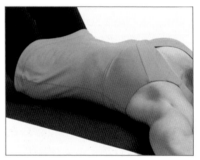

Strong abs prevent the back from arching or sagging.

Be sure to support your neck on moves that ask you to clasp your hands behind your head, like the Diamond Crunch and the Double Bicycle, and resist the temptation to close your elbows together and yank up. Instead, round your elbows outward, relax your shoulders, and hold that shape. Your hands are there only for support; your abs should do all the heavy lifting—no yanking or pulling on your head (it won't make things easier anyway).

And don't forget proper breathing, perhaps the most neglected aspect of core training. By exhaling strongly through your mouth as you exert an effort and inhaling through your mouth as you release the effort, you work deep transverse muscle fibers that would not otherwise get into the act.

Follow these rules to change your midsection in noticeable, significant ways in just a few short weeks, especially if you consistently focus on giving it your all for 10 minutes.

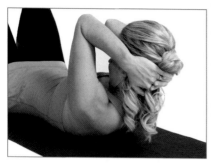

This is a no-no!

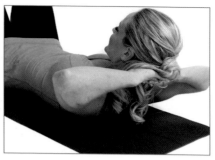

This is the right way to do it: Keep your elbows wide and shoulders relaxed.

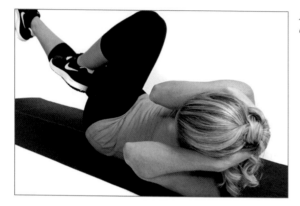

Avoid this common mistake on your bicycle crunches!

CORE & MORE WORKOUT

Keep in Mind
- follow the weekly recommendations for this workout based on the exercise level you chose in chapter 2
- the main focus is on strengthening and sculpting core muscles

What You Need
- an exercise mat or thick bath towel or rug

What to Expect
- to burn about seventy-five calories

Set Time Chart

Bracing Bridges	1 minute	Elbow-Plank Walks	1 minute
Diamond Crunch	1 minute	Side-Plank Knee Lift	2 minutes
Hip Lifts	1 minute	Cobra Reach	1 minute
Double Bicycle	1 minute	Crawling Plank	1 minute
X Out 'n' In	1 minute	**TOTAL TIME**	**10 MINUTES**

Interval 1
Bracing Bridges
(1 minute)

Start: Lie on your back with both knees bent, feet flat on the mat and hip width apart, and toes pointing straight ahead. Rest your arms on the mat along your sides, palms down. Relax your head and shoulders.

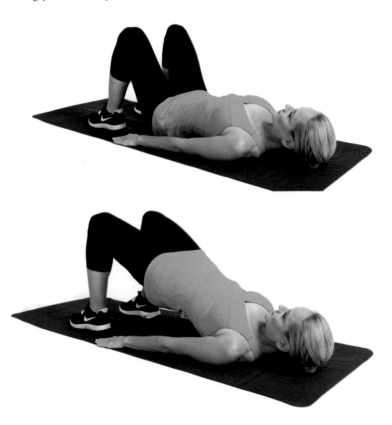

Move: Inhale deeply through your nose. As you exhale through your mouth, brace your belly button into your spine, and lift your hips off the mat so that your tailbone points toward the ceiling, keeping knees bent and pointing straight ahead over your toes. Hold bridge for three counts and then slowly lower your hips to the mat.

That's one rep. Repeat as many times as you can for 1 minute, focusing on connecting your breath with the contraction of your abdominals and on using your core muscles rather than your legs to power your hip movement.

Ⓢimplify It:

Rather than lifting your hips high off the mat, simply brace your abdominals and tilt your pelvis slightly so your tailbone and buttocks lift off the mat but your back remains stationary.

Ⓐdvance It:

For a greater balance and core challenge, alternate lifting your feet an inch or so off the mat as you lift your hips into the bridge.

Anywhere Abs

Whenever you have a little time to "waist," sneak in these moves to strengthen your core, ease back pain, and improve posture:

In your chair. Sit up tall with your back away from the backrest and your feet flat on the floor. Raise your arms and clasp your hands together. Keeping your abs tight, lean to the left as far as you can, hold for ten slow counts, and then return to center. Alternate left and right leans for ten on each side. Remember to keep breathing.

On your feet. Stand tall with a long, relaxed spine and brace your abdominal muscles by taking a breath, strongly tightening your ab muscles and holding for ten slow counts. Focus on tightening the deeper muscles several layers down. Repeat ten times or more.

On the bus or train. When you're on the bus or train, grab the overhead rail with one or both hands and tense your arm as if you're doing a pull-up. At the same time, press your feet into the floor. Use your core muscles to "fight" these opposing forces for ten slow counts. Repeat ten or more times.

Interval 2
Diamond Crunch
(1 minute)

Start: Lie on your back with your head and shoulders resting on the mat. Clasp your hands behind your head and open your arms out to the sides, with your elbows bent. Lift your feet off the mat, press your heels together, and drop your bent knees out to the side so your legs form a diamond shape.

Move: Inhale deeply through your mouth and lower your legs about halfway to the floor, maintaining the diamond shape and keeping your lower back in contact with the mat—that is, don't arch your back. Exhale and draw your abdominals in tightly as you rock your legs back toward your body while simultaneously lifting your head and shoulders up and forward toward your legs. Lower your legs and head back to start position.

That's one rep. Repeat as many times as you can for 1 minute. Maintain good form and move slowly and with purpose to avoid using too much momentum.

Simplify It:

Instead of lifting and lowering your legs, keep your knees bent and relax your knees to the sides as you press the soles of your feet together. Just perform the upper body part of the crunch.

Advance It:

As you lower your legs toward the floor, straighten both legs and lower them until they are parallel to the ground—remember, don't arch your back—squeezing your inner thighs and the sides of your knees together. Bend both knees back into the diamond shape again as you lift into crunch position.

Interval 3
Hip Lifts
(1 minute)

Start: Lie on your back with arms relaxed at your sides, palms down, head and shoulders resting on the mat. Extend your legs up over your hips, keeping them as straight as your flexibility comfortably allows and press your heels toward the ceiling.

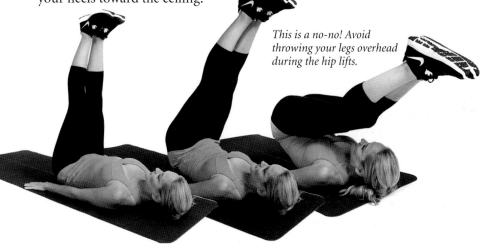

This is a no-no! Avoid throwing your legs overhead during the hip lifts.

Move: Inhale deeply through your nose. Then exhale through your mouth as you press your arms into the mat and tilt your pelvis up and forward so that your hips are lifted a bit off the floor. Hold for one count, and then slowly lower your hips back to the mat. Power this move from your core rather than swinging your legs to build up momentum.

That's one rep. Do as many repetitions as you can, with good form, for 1 minute.

Simplify It:

Instead of lifting your hips off the mat, just focus on tilting your pelvis up and scooping your abdominals into your back.

Advance It:

Lift both arms a few inches off the mat and extend them straight back behind you so they are alongside your ears.

Flat-Belly Myths

A guaranteed flat-belly cure is as sought after as a cure for the common cold—such a bummer that neither exists. With all manner of pills, potions, and programs declaring they magically melt the fat off your middle, watch out for the following three belly-busting scams:

Flat-Belly Zappers. Gadgets that claim to zap the fat off your middle with electric shocks have been around for more than a century. The problem is that electricity doesn't do anything to budge belly fat. The only thing these doodads lighten up is your wallet. The verdict? Skip it. Want an instant way to help flatten your belly? Try the "drawing-in maneuver" anytime, anywhere: Sit (or stand) tall, and draw your bellybutton in toward your spine, bracing your abdominals into your back but still allowing yourself to breathe comfortably. Hold for 10 seconds; then relax. Build up to holding for 30 seconds at a time—while in traffic or at your desk, in line at the bank, or anywhere else—to flatten your belly.

Fat-Burning Foods. Snacking your way to a taut tummy is right up there with unicorns and fairies on the "things we wish were true but aren't" list. No food we know of targets stomach fat for extinction, but there's plenty of evidence that burning more calories than you eat does. Instead of trying to find a magic food, focus on filling your belly with fiber. Eating whole, naturally fiber-filled foods like pears, avocados, artichokes, and lentils is not only nutritious, it may also help you stay fuller, longer (which means you have less room for junk). Plus, fiber helps keep things moving along in your digestive system, which can mean less bloat and puffiness.

Tummy-Toning Pills. Looking for the scientific proof that supplements shrink your tummy without diet and exercise? There isn't any. Not a shred of evidence. If all it took were a pill, we'd all be taking it. Want an easier, less expensive, and more effective alternative to diet pills? Water! A recent Virginia Tech study found that when overweight adults on a diet drank 16 ounces of water a half hour before every meal for twelve weeks, they lost almost five pounds more than those who didn't.[15] Why? Water helps you feel full, which can lead you to consume fewer calories at mealtimes. Be sure to allow enough time for it to work, so drink up about 10–15 minutes before eating.

Interval 4

Double Bicycle
(1 minute)

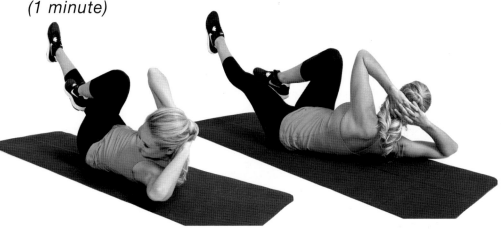

Start: Lie on your back with your head and shoulders resting on the mat. Clasp your hands together behind your head and open your arms out to the sides, with your elbows bent. Bend your knees, lift your feet off the mat, and draw your knees into your chest.

Move: Keeping your right knee drawn into your chest, extend your left leg out straight and parallel to the floor. Lift both shoulders off the mat and, twisting from your core, move your left shoulder toward your right knee. (Keep your elbows rounded rather than pulling on your neck to move.) Pulse your shoulder toward the knee twice; then twist through your core to switch your arm and leg positions.

That's one rep. Do as many repetitions as you can, with good form, alternating sides each time for 1 minute.

Ⓢimplify It:

Extend your raised leg at a 45-degree angle to the floor or higher.

Ⓐdvance It:

Extend both legs out straight and parallel to the floor. Then, as you twist your left shoulder across, bend your right knee in and hold for pulses. Straighten your right leg out again so that both legs are extended as you switch sides.

Interval 5
X Out 'n' In
(1 minute)

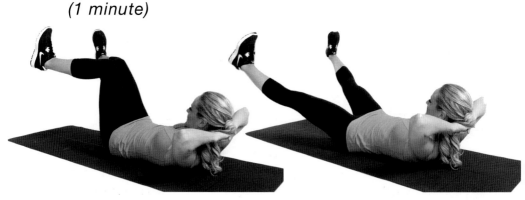

Start: Lie on your back with both hands clasped together behind your head, elbows bent and open to the sides. Lift your head and shoulders off the mat and lift your feet so your knees are bent at a 90-degree angle above your hips. Flex your feet and press the insides of your knees together so that your heels turn out.

Move: Keeping your head and shoulders lifted, draw in your abdominals and press out through your heels to separate your legs and extend them straight out toward the corners of your mat. Hold for one count, and then bend your knees in, returning your legs to start position. (Keep your head up the entire time.) Focus on keeping your pelvis parallel to the floor as you move your legs, making sure not to arch or completely flatten your lower back into the mat.

That's one rep. Repeat as many times as you can for 1 minute.

(S)implify It:

Keep your head and shoulders on the mat, and just perform the leg movements.

(A)dvance It:

Keeping your head and shoulders lifted off the ground, extend your arms out straight and back by your ears, with your palms facing up.

Interval 6

Elbow-Plank Walks
(1 minute)

Start: Lie facedown on the mat with your legs out straight and arms bent, elbows under your shoulders and palms pressed against the mat. Lift your body off the mat so you are propped up on your elbows and the underside of your toes and so your spine forms a straight line from the top of your head to your heels. Tighten your core so your back neither sags nor arches.

Move: Keeping your body in a straight line, alternate moving your feet to "walk" your toes out until your legs are outside your hips, and then walk them back to the start position.

That's one rep. Repeat as many times as you can for 1 minute.

Simplify It:

Slow the pace as much as possible. Rest during the minute, if necessary, coming down to your knees if needed.

Advance It:

Instead of "walking" your feet apart and together, "jump" them apart and then together, making sure your hips don't pop up higher than shoulder level.

Interval 7
Side-Plank Knee Lift
(2 minutes)

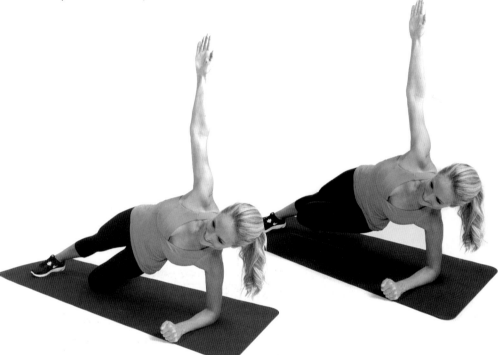

Start: Lie on your left side, propped up on your left forearm and with your hips stacked directly on top of each other. Then extend your right arm directly above your shoulder, palm facing away from you. Straighten your right leg and bend your left knee so that your foot is behind you. Pull your abs in and lift your torso off the floor so you're balanced on your left forearm and the inside of your right foot and your bent left leg is resting on the floor.

Move: Holding your body in this side-plank position, lift your left knee off the floor and move it forward until your left foot is directly beneath the inside of your right knee. Press your foot into your knee and squeeze your inner thighs together, holding for one count; then lower your left leg back to the start position. As you move your left leg, keep the rest of your body as still and as stable as possible and your abdominals braced into your back.

That's one rep. Repeat as many times as you can for 1 minute. Then turn onto your right side and repeat for 1 minute.

(S)implify It:

Keep your left knee on the mat the whole time and simply work on holding the side-plank position for up to 1 minute. Take breaks, if needed, by lowering your hips to the mat.

(A)dvance It:

Keep your left knee lifted and your left foot pressed into the right leg the entire time. And instead of lifting and lowering your left leg, turn your left knee toward the ceiling, crossing the midline of your body, and then bring it back in line with your hip. As you turn your knee in and out, be sure to keep your hips square and your pelvis steady.

Burst Your Bubbles

Not all of the roundness in your tummy can be chalked up to extra pudge. Some of it may be due to gassiness, so in your effort to achieve a flat belly, avoid foods that give you serious gas. That means skipping carbonated drinks, including diet sodas. Regular soda is just empty calories, but the artificial sweeteners combined with the bubbles in diet soda can inflate the stomach like a balloon. Also, diet soda is now being linked to larger waistlines. One University of Texas study found that, over a twelve-year period, people who drank two or more diet sodas a day experienced waist size increases that were five times greater than people who did not drink diet soda.[16] Your best bet is to avoid fizzy drinks altogether and stick with plain old water. If you need to quickly reduce some bloat, try squeezing a little lemon or lime in your water. It adds flavor and is a natural mild diuretic that can help flush out excess fluid right before a big event or a swimsuit debut.

Interval 8
Cobra Reach
(1 minute)

Start: Lie facedown on
the mat with your legs out
straight, hip width apart, heels up,
and the underside of your toes pressing into
the mat. Bend your arms and place your elbows underneath your shoulders, palms facing down and chest resting on the mat.

Move: Arch your back gently and lift your head, shoulders, and chest off
the mat. Be careful not to press with your arms to lift. Keep your legs on the
mat. As you lift your chest, extend your right arm straight in front of you
alongside your right ear, palm down. Keep your chin tucked into your chest
and your eyes looking down. Lower your chest to the mat as you bend your
right elbow in and return to start position. Repeat with the left arm.

That's one rep. Repeat as many times as you can for 1 minute.

(S)implify It:

Instead of extending your arms, keep them bent and resting on the mat
as you gently arch your back to lift your chest.

(A)dvance It:

Instead of alternating your arms, lift both arms off the mat as you extend
your spine and then bend both in to the mat as you lower your chest.

Interval 9
Crawling Plank
(1 minute)

Start: Kneel down so that your knees are aligned beneath your hips and your palms are aligned beneath your shoulders. Draw your abdominals up and into your back and then, keeping your spine in a straight line, lift your knees a few inches off the mat, being careful not to lift your hips.

Move: Keep your spine straight and your core strong as you alternate your hands to walk them forward, twice each hand, to move into an extended plank, hands a few inches in front of your shoulders. Reverse directions and walk your hands back to the start position. Make sure your hips don't pop up above shoulder level and don't let your back sag.

That's one rep. Repeat as many times as you can for 1 minute.

Ⓢimplify It:

Keep your knees bent and lightly touching the ground for more support in your plank position. Walk your hands out while maintaining this modified plank position.

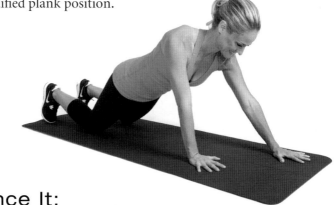

Ⓐdvance It:

Instead of keeping both feet on the floor during the crawl, lift your right foot off the floor, and extend your right leg straight behind your hip. Keep your right leg in this position as you walk your hands out and then back in, switching legs before repeating on the other side. Alternate legs each time.

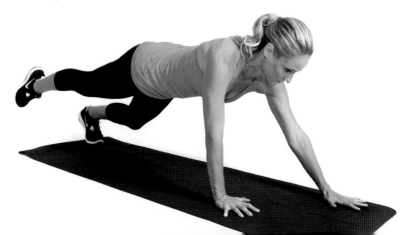

The Thin in 10 Advantage:
Lose This Fat

It's true that no food makes the fat around your midsection disappear, but one additive does seem to make it appear faster. Trans fat—an ingredient commonly found in foods such as margarines, crackers, and baked goods—has been shown to promote abdominal fat deposits. When Wake Forest University School of Medicine researchers in North Carolina fed monkeys large amounts of these unhealthy fats, the critters deposited 30 percent more blubber around their abdomens than the monkeys subsisting on a healthier diet free of trans fats.[17] So one real *Thin in 10* advantage? Our diet plan is complete with recipes that minimize your intake of trans fats.

Wrap-Up

Our testers consistently commented that they could feel their core muscles working as they did this workout. We're not surprised to hear it. We chose this particular combination of moves because it attacks your core from every angle. Try this workout for yourself. Don't waste time on longer core workouts when this compact routine does its job so well. The Core Conditioning DVD workout gets the job done too.

7 | The 10-Minute Stretch

"I look forward to this 'stretch break' more than anything else during the day!"
—Suzanne, original *Thin in 10* focus group member

Believe it or not, the act of bending over to touch your toes has turned out to be one of the most controversial fitness topics. That's because stretching doesn't appear to offer all the benefits we once thought. It doesn't help that expert advice about stretching is all over the place. Should you stretch before a workout? Should you stretch afterward? Should you bother stretching at all? In this chapter, we sort fact from fiction and then explain why stretching is an essential part of the *Thin in 10* plan.

Stretching, the Truth

For decades, stretching before a workout to prevent injury and soreness was one of the golden rules. Then, to avoid stretching muscles when they are at their coldest and tightest, experts started recommending stretching at the end of a workout or at least waiting until after a sufficient warm-up. In 2001, a research retrospective commissioned by the IDEA Health & Fitness Association challenged many of these ideas about stretching.[18]

The report, an extensive review of dozens of studies, found that stretching does not prevent injuries—whether it's done before, during, or after a workout—and may actually increase the risk of injury by making the joints less stable. Injury risk also spikes if you stretch incorrectly or push a muscle too far. The pre-workout stretch seems to leave joints especially vulnerable because that's when muscles and tendons are cold and more likely to strain or tear. The same report showed that stretching doesn't lessen the suffering related to post-workout muscle soreness either. In addition, it may have a negative impact on both strength and athletic performance; several studies in the retrospective found that weight lifters who stretch between sets actually have less strength to finish their workouts. The research is mixed about whether stretching relieves back pain. Even though back stretches are a staple in most back pain programs, some investigations have found that stretching decreases range of motion and makes the situation worse.

Although stretching might not be of much use for preventing injury or soreness, we still believe it has value overall. We'd like to reframe the purpose of stretching and explain how it benefits flexibility.

Why We Stretch

The simple truth is that you look better when you're more flexible. When your muscles are relaxed, you appear more lengthened. Being limber helps you stand up straighter so you have better posture and move more gracefully. People who are obviously stiff shuffle along with rounded shoulders. Besides looking as if they're in pain, they're at greater risk for losing their balance and falling. They also lack what scientists call normal range of motion.

When a joint has normal range of motion, it's able to easily move the way it needs to in order to do its job. To understand how important having a normal range of motion is, think about reaching up for a sweater on the top shelf of a closet or twisting around in the front seat of your car for your purse on the backseat. Without decent flexibility, these basic, everyday actions become challenging tasks and may even lead to injury.

And while many studies have disputed its benefits, stretching may still improve your strength if you get your timing down. A recent study published in the *Journal of Strength and Conditioning Research* found that subjects who did strength training three times a week, followed by two stretching sessions, tripled their muscle strength when compared to those who skipped stretching or stretched between sets.[19] As noted, stretching—like lifting—causes tiny tears in your muscle and as your body repairs them, the tissue becomes stronger.

Also, don't underestimate the power of stretching to help you chill out. This is no small thing considering the multitasking, overproductive, stressed-out world in which we live. When surveyed, people who stretch report feeling more energetic and focused, yet calmer. Gentle stretching sends a message to the nervous system, telling your adrenal glands to limit their release of the stress hormones adrenaline and cortisol, a particularly troublesome hormone associated with both increased blood sugar and storage of belly fat. A good amount of evidence shows how the act of stretching increases blood flow into common stress-holding areas like the neck and shoulders, making them feel less tight and tense. This prevents and alleviates chronic stress-related conditions such as neck pain, headaches, and carpal tunnel syndrome. Ever notice how stress relief is promoted as a huge benefit of yoga and Pilates? This is why.

> "People who stretch report feeling more energetic and focused, yet calmer."

Stretching just before bed is also a great way to unwind and release your day. Stretching just before bed may help you sleep more soundly, as one of our focus group members reported. It's up to you to decide when to stretch, but we highly recommend looking at this activity as an opportunity to help lower belly fat-inducing cortisol levels, one stretch at a time.

We also contend that while everybody needs some flexibility, they need the right amount of flexibility for what they do. It seems obvious that prima ballerinas and Olympic gymnasts use flexibility differently than runners or tennis players do—or the average person. A dancer with the flexibility of a runner is going to be so tight that she risks pulling a muscle the first time she tries a *rond de jambe*, while a marathoner with the flexibility of a dancer is going to be so loose her joints will be less stable, increasing her risk for an injury. (Studies prove this, by the way.)

In other words, some people require more flexibility to perform at the top of their game than others. It makes perfect sense, then, to work toward the optimum amount of flexibility you need to perform your personal best. If your goal is to do a complete back bend, obviously you've got to dedicate more time to stretching than someone who simply wants to feel better. The stretching program we've designed is aimed at improving posture and fluidity of movement and helping you de-stress. It's gentle enough to sidestep many of the negatives of stretching we referenced earlier. We believe it's the ideal routine for anyone working on their *Thin in 10* transformation.

How to Stretch

There are several styles of stretching, and all of them can work very well for improving flexibility and helping you feel better. Our program is based on the theory of static stretching, the kind recommended by the American College of Sports Medicine and many other professional fitness organizations. However, we also encourage you to give other stretching styles, such as active isolated stretching, a try if you want to make flexibility one of your main priorities. Static stretching calls for you to warm up to increase blood flow and raise body temperature to the working muscle. We do this as a safety precaution— and because stretching a muscle that's tight and stiff is no fun. Our stretching routine begins with a quick warm-up and then gently eases into more intensive stretches for safety. Alternatively, you can do the stretching routine right after you've completed one of the other *Thin in 10* workouts.

Always start out slowly and carefully. Your first repetition of a stretch may not take you that far or you may be gradually able to move into a longer stretch as you hold the position. Once you move into a stretch position to your point of comfort, hold it for 30 seconds; use one of the timers we recommend in chapter 4, "Cardio QUICK," or count slowly to twenty. As you move into a stretch, inhale deeply through your nose; as you move out of the stretch, exhale strongly through your mouth. A good steady breath increases oxygen and blood flow into the working muscle and promotes relaxation.

When coming out of a stretch, release the position carefully. If there's no pain or undue tightness, repeat it again. Be sure not to bounce forcefully or push, snap, or jerk your muscles into position. When you stretch a muscle on the right side, be sure to stretch the left side too. The same goes for opposing muscle groups: When you stretch a muscle attached to the front of the joint, you should give equal time to the muscle attached to the back. If you feel a sharp pain or something doesn't otherwise feel right, back off on the stretch to see if that helps. Or try the modified version we suggest. If it still hurts, accept that this is not an exercise for you and move on.

If you're seriously inflexible, that's okay. You're here to make improvements so don't feel discouraged. Consider using a towel or belt to extend your reach for stretch positions that are beyond you at the moment. The primary focus during this routine is to stretch not only your body but also your mind. Look at this as a time-out from your day. Emphasize breathing, relaxing, and clearing your mind versus trying to "perform" during this session.

> "When you stretch a muscle on the right side, be sure to stretch the left side too."

THE 10-MINUTE STRETCH WORKOUT

Keep in Mind
- follow the weekly recommendations for this workout based on the exercise level you chose in chapter 2, but know that you can choose to do this session up to seven days a week for its relaxation and calming benefits

What You Need
- mat or a thick towel (optional)

What to Expect
- to feel looser, more relaxed, and able to move more fluidly
- over time, to feel that way most of the time

Set Time Chart

Wake-Up	1 minute
Standing Side Stretch	30 seconds
Chest/Back Opener	30 seconds
Cat/Cow	1 minute
Back Extensions	1 minute
Child's Pose Side Stretch	1 minute (30/30)
Prone Quad Stretch	1 minute (30/30)
Seated Hurdler's Stretch	1 minute (30/30)
Seated Spine Twist	1 minute (30/30)
Butterfly Stretch	1 minute
Supine Lower Back	1 minute
TOTAL TIME	**10 MINUTES**

Wake-Up

High-Knee Marches
in Place

(1 minute)

Interval 1

Standing Side Stretch

(30 seconds)

Start: Stand tall and relaxed with your feet together. Reach both arms overhead toward the ceiling and clasp the back of one hand in the other.

Stretch: Take a deep breath in and, as you exhale, reach your arms even farther and lean to the right. Stretch as far to the side as you comfortably can, pressing your left hip out slightly to increase the stretch. Inhale and return to the start position; then exhale and repeat the stretch to the left. Repeat this slowly and carefully as many times as you can for 30 seconds.

Interval 2
Chest/Back Opener
(30 seconds)

Start: Stand tall and relaxed with your feet together. Raise your arms out in front of you at chest level and clasp your hands together. Round your elbows slightly and press your palms away from you.

Stretch: Inhale and press your arms away from your body as you hollow your abdomen, round your upper body, and release your chin toward your chest. Hold the stretch and breathe easily for 15 seconds. Next, clasp your hands together behind your back, interlacing your fingers and extending your arms as high up as you can without collapsing through your chest. Keep your chest lifted and chin slightly up. Hold and breathe for 15 seconds.

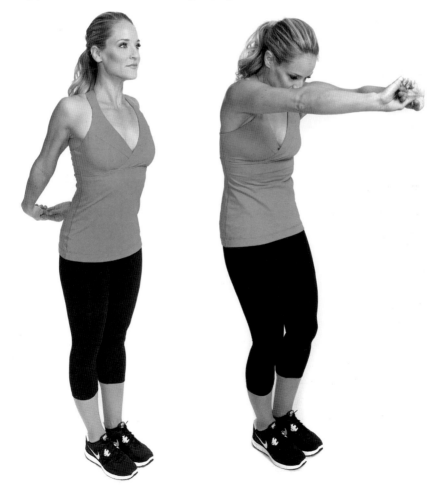

Interval 3
Cat/Cow
(1 minute)

Start: Kneel on the floor (on a mat or towel if you wish to cushion your joints), placing your hands directly under your shoulders and your knees directly under your hips.

Stretch: Inhale. Round your back and curl your chin toward your chest, tucking your tailbone under. Next, exhale slowly and arch your back, looking up to the ceiling and releasing your belly to the floor; avoid sinking into your shoulders. Flow slowly, gently, and continually through this movement, following the natural rhythm of your breath, for 1 minute.

Interval 4
Back Extensions
(1 minute)

Start: Lie facedown, with your legs extended straight out behind you, elbows bent, and palms pressed into the floor in front of your shoulders.
Stretch: Inhale deeply. Then, as you exhale, gently press away from the floor, extending your spine to lift your chest and abdomen (but not your hips) off the floor. Keep your shoulders down and back and lift through your sternum. Hold for one or two counts and then gently release back to the floor. Repeat slowly, smoothly, and continually for 1 minute.

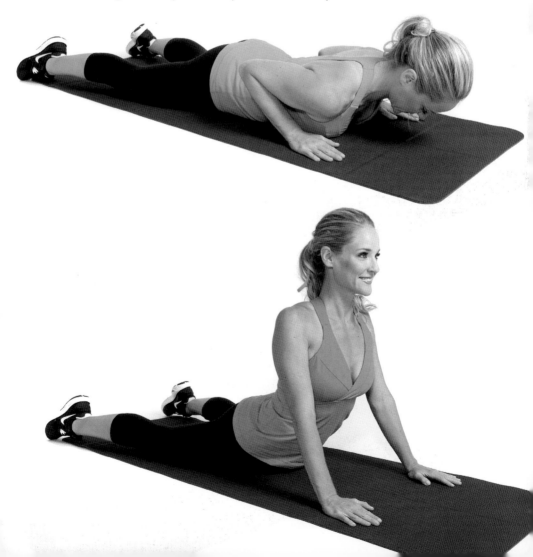

Interval 5
Child's Pose Side Stretch
(1 minute)

Start: Kneel down on all fours with the tops of your feet relaxed (don't tuck your toes under). Gently lower your buttocks back, sitting as close to the back of your heels as you comfortably can. Rest your chest over your thighs and reach your arms out on the floor in front of your body, head down and relaxed, eyes looking toward the floor.

Stretch: Keeping your head down and hips back on your heels, slowly walk both hands over to the right side, stretching through the left side of your torso as you go. Hold and breathe for 30 seconds; then slowly walk over to the left side and repeat for 30 seconds.

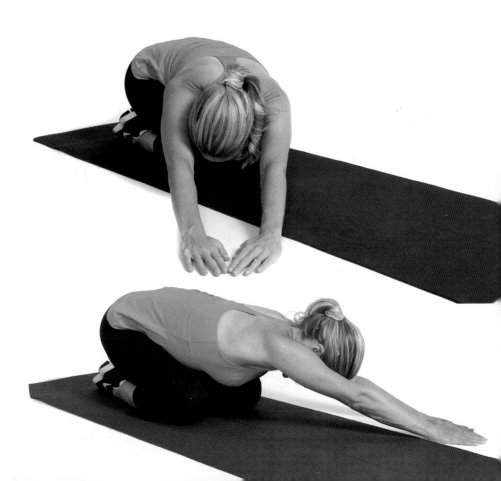

Interval 6
Prone Quad Stretch
(1 minute)

Start: Lie facedown with your arms resting on the floor, elbows bent and open to the sides, palms stacked on top of each other, and your forehead resting on the backs of your hands. Extend your legs straight out behind you, with the tops of your feet resting on the floor.

Stretch: Bend your right knee and bring your heel toward your body. Reach back with your right hand and grab your right ankle. Gently draw in your right heel as close to your body as you comfortably can, while pressing your hips forward into the floor. Hold for 30 seconds, taking deep relaxing breaths and then switch to the left side and hold for 30 seconds. Note: If you aren't able to grab your ankle in this position, try this in a side-lying position instead.

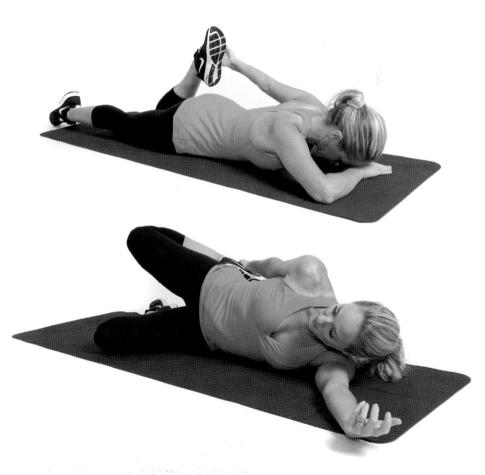

Interval 7
Seated Hurdler's Stretch
(1 minute)

Start: Sit on the floor with your legs extended straight out in front of you. Bend your left knee and place the sole of your left foot as high on the inside of your right thigh as your flexibility comfortably allows.

Stretch: Hinge forward from your hips, and reach both arms out, stretching your fingertips as close to your right foot as you can (if you are able to, hold on to your foot with both hands). Avoid excessively rounding your back and try to bring your chest as close to your thighs as possible. Hold this position for 30 seconds, breathing comfortably. Switch legs and repeat for 30 seconds.

One Recommendation That's All Wet

The myth that you must drink eight, eight-ounce glasses of water has finally drowned under its own weight. A review from the prestigious *Journal of the American Society of Nephrology* specifically addressed this issue and found no real basis—and more important, no real health benefits—for the recommendation.

Of course, it's important to get adequate fluid intake from liquids and juicy foods, especially when it's hot and when you exercise. We think water is the healthiest choice of beverages. Is it as fun as soda, or juice, or a sports drink? Nah. But it's not packed with calories or chemicals that may be bad for your health either.

Interval 8

Seated Spine Twist

(1 minute)

Start: Sit on the floor with your left leg extended straight out in front of you. Step your right foot over your extended left leg and pull your right leg gently toward your chest so that your right knee is pointing toward the ceiling.

Stretch: Place your right hand on the floor just behind your right hip. Sit up as tall as you can and twist through your waist until you are looking over your right shoulder and feel a stretch spread through your hips. Hold and breathe for 30 seconds and then repeat to the other side for 30 seconds.

The *Thin in 10* Advantage:

Simplicity

This 10-minute session is simple! While we love yoga and Pilates for their great flexibility and relaxation benefits, they can carry a hefty learning curve before you experience any mind-body payoffs. We purposely kept our stretch routine simple and straightforward. We wanted it to be doable without your having to worry about how to practice the "uddiyan bandha" technique, as you might be asked to do in a yoga class. Think about this session as a time-out for your body and mind—you should finish feeling restored, energized, and maybe a little looser.

Interval 9
Butterfly Stretch
(1 minute)

Start: Sit on the floor with the soles of your feet together
and your knees bent and open out to the sides.
Stretch: Grasp your ankles with both hands and gently
hinge forward from your hips, bringing your chest as
close to your feet as possible. For a greater stretch,
press your elbows down gently onto the insides
of your knees to open your legs farther. Be cau-
tious not to push too far or round your back
too much. Hold for 1 minute.

Interval 10
Supine Lower Back
(1 minute)

Start: Lie on your back.
Stretch: Bend both of your knees and draw them
into your chest. Hug your lower legs with both hands to draw
your knees closer to your chest. Relax your neck and shoulders, pressing your lower back wide into the floor, keeping your tailbone down. Hold
for 1 minute, taking deep relaxing breaths.

Stretching the Heartstrings

Can stretching your muscles also make your arteries more flexible? According to scientists at the University of North Texas, it's entirely possible. The researchers asked more than 500 participants of both genders and all ages to do a "sit and reach" stretch very similar to the hurdler stretch in our stretch routine.[20] As subjects reached for their toes, their blood pressure was measured using cuffs attached to both their arms and legs. Since blood pressure provides an indication of how flexible the arteries are and how freely blood can flow through the entire cardiovascular system, it's often used to assess risk of heart attack and stroke.

To the researchers' amazement, they uncovered a strong association between flexible bodies and flexible arteries in all the subjects over forty (not so in the younger crowd, however). Add to this a smaller, older University of Austin study, which found that stretching increases arterial flexibility by nearly 20 percent and you have the basis for an intriguing theory: Stretching is good for your heart! Of course, no one is suggesting that if you have trouble bending down to tie your shoes you're on the fast track to heart trouble. While stiffer arteries do indicate a less efficient heart, the current evidence doesn't imply that you can stretch your way around a heart attack. Still, it's certainly a subject that deserves further study. In the meantime, keep stretching to enjoy the many other benefits.

Wrap-Up

Think of this stretching routine as our version of stopping to smell the roses. Testers told us they could feel the tension in their muscles melt away when they did this stretch workout. Try it yourself to understand what they're talking about. Or feel free to swap in the Stretch & De-stress DVD workout for a similar experience. Remember to take deep breaths, allow yourself to relax, and indulge in these 10 minutes of "me time." You're worth it.

PART II

The *Thin in 10* Meal Plan

8 | Your 10-Minutes-or-Less Meal Plan

We know you're busy. We know eating right can be a challenge. We also know that you probably think eating healthy involves creating a lengthy grocery list and enduring an even more arduous cooking process. None of this is true with the *Thin in 10* meal plan. This time you really can toss that "but I don't have time to eat healthy" excuse out the window.

The next four chapters include fabulous recipes for breakfast, lunch, dinner, and an optional snack or dessert. All of the recipes are delicious yet simple enough for even less experienced cooks to make. And, as we're about to explain, taking the time to prepare these recipes is the foundation of the *Thin in 10* eating plan.

From this point forward, we ask you to prepare the majority of your own meals. For some of you, this is an important lifestyle modification. It means eating no more than one to three meals outside the home, which means eating at home at least six days a week. You may view this as a huge, unnecessary inconvenience. If so, consider the research: Eating out frequently has been directly linked to having a higher body mass index (BMI) and body fat percentage. One study found that women who eat out more than five times a week consume, on average, 290 calories more per day than those who stay in and cook.

These findings aren't terribly surprising when you consider that the Center for Science in the Public Interest found most restaurant meals are at least double—and in many cases triple—the recommended serving size. Takeout dinners are a diet land mine too. You're likely to eat 131 percent more with takeout compared to a meal you prepare yourself, according to one study.

All the Advantages

Perhaps you cook on a regular basis; perhaps you don't. If you avoid cooking because it's either stressful or time-consuming, we understand. We used to feel the same way. But our recipes are so quick and easy they can be prepared by anyone. Even novices can pull them off. Every single one of our recipes can be made in about 10 minutes or less. Cleanup isn't too bad either; plus this burns extra calories! The planning, prep, and minimal shopping needed actually take less time than waiting for a pizza delivery—and the end result is a tasty, healthy meal. And as for you chefs out there, these recipes are so delicious, they'll satisfy your taste buds too. For those times you must eat out—no more than once a week, please—stick with our list of "eating on the go" options to avoid blowing all of your hard work.

"Our recipes are so quick and easy they can be prepared by anyone."

Making your own meals is also significantly less expensive than getting takeout or dining out. By following this plan, your wallet gets less of a workout and probably will get fatter as you get thinner. Plus, we've made sure to include ingredients that won't break the bank; as one tester, Keri, put it, "I love that I can use frozen produce—I can usually get store-bought brands for $1." And, as we said, whipping up these recipes usually takes less time than waiting for your meal to be delivered.

If you've already been preparing your own meals regularly, our plan supports you and helps you stick with choices that are lean and healthy.

A Better Shopping Experience

Going to the grocery store when you are tight on time can be a nightmare. The following tips can make your experience a little less hectic (and cheaper too):

Don't shop the ends of aisles. Stores display the products they want to sell the most of at either end of an aisle because they know you are more likely to see these items and grab one as you round the corner. Usually these are packaged, nonessential items that you, your pocketbook, and your diet can live without.

Shop the perimeter of the store. Countless nutrition experts offer this advice—and for good reason. The outer edges of the store contain fresh and frozen produce, meats, and dairy products. The deeper into the center of the store you go, the more packaged and processed the foods become.

Shop on Tuesdays. Many surveys name Tuesday as the least crowded day of the week. Most deliveries are made early in the week so produce is fresher on Tuesday.

Save by squatting down. Stores line the shelves from top to bottom in order of price. The top, eye-level products—often referred to as the "thigh to eye" line—are usually the priciest. Squat down to peer at the bottom shelf to find a similar item for a lower price.

Get your turkey on first. Shopping when you're hungry is a recipe for disaster. All the smells and sights in the store are hard to resist if your stomach is rumbling. One study found that eating foods rich in tryptophan (such as turkey) can help raise levels of the feel-good brain chemical serotonin and lower your urge to spend.

Carry a basket. Carrying a basket makes it easier to move through the store faster and decreases your chances of tossing in unnecessary items. Plus, faster movements burn more calories.

Grocery lists? Yeah, there are aps for that—Grocery IQ for the iPhone (http://bit.ly/Sd2Vk0) or Grocery Gadget for other smart phones (http://bit.ly/s4ruZB). Of course, you can also create a grocery list the old-fashioned way—with pen and paper.

All of our *Thin in 10* recipes were created especially for this plan by registered dietitian Lauren O'Connor (owner of Nutri-Savvy in Los Angeles and a busy mom of twin toddlers) and meet our recommended nutritional and weight-loss guidelines. We don't ask you to embrace the idea of eating tofu and seaweed. We worked with Lauren to ensure that the ingredients we use are simple, wholesome, and found in any market; we promise not to send you down some exotic food aisle searching for an expensive product whose name you can't pronounce and that no one likes the taste of.

Easy as 1-2-3

To guarantee our plan supports your weight-loss efforts, we've done the math. Our diet is based on 1,500 calories a day. This assumes you are a woman who wants to lose weight; men might consider bumping their calorie count up to 1,800–2,100 calories per day to account for differences in the male metabolism. However, there's no calorie counting involved, so you can just follow the recipes without checking any charts or busting out a calculator. It works like this:

All breakfast recipes are 300 calories or less (chapter 9).
All lunch recipes are 400 calories or less (chapter 10).
All dinner recipes are 600 calories or less (chapter 11).
Choose from snack suggestions for an additional 200 calories (chapter 12).

All you need to do is follow the guidelines for each of the meal categories every day. Stick with that idea to eat about 1,500 calories a day—enough so you can lose weight without feeling deprived. Note that all of

Avoiding Allergens

Food allergies or intolerances can be a dangerous problem for some people. The last thing we want is to advise you to use an ingredient that will make you sick or worse. If you encounter an ingredient in a recipe that you are allergic to, simply use the substitution you normally use or ask your medical care provider for a suitable alternative. Don't let allergies stop you from finding new, healthy recipes.

Is Your Healthy Food Bland?

Some of the biggest culprits responsible for weight gain—sugar, sodium, and unhealthy fats—add rich, satisfying flavor to foods. When weaning yourself off highly processed foods, everything may taste kind of, well, blah. It can take a few weeks to cleanse your palate to enjoy the clean flavors of a more natural, health-conscious menu.

Lauren recommends giving your taste buds a lift in the following ways:

1. *Use healthy spices.* Add spices and herbs such as basil, chili powder, garlic, or onion to liven up beef dishes. For chicken, try bay leaf, rosemary, or marjoram. Zip up the taste of fish with a splash of citrus, and use a dash of sage, rosemary, or thyme on pork. You can even experiment with inspired spice combos on eggs, potatoes, and veggies. Don't be afraid to mix it up in new ways.

2. *Try some premixed seasonings.* Mrs. Dash offers some tasty spice mixes designed for specific meats and types of cooking. Just make sure the blend you choose is a no- or low-sodium version.

3. *Hummus makes a great mayonnaise substitute.* Try a flavor that's been spiked with citrus, garlic, or spice. This is a surprisingly simple, low-calorie way of adding a kick to your cooking.

4. *Chop up the protein in your dish into smaller morsels.* That way you get more taste per square inch.

our recipes are for single servings. When feeding your family, simply multiply your ingredients by the number of people eating and stick to serving sizes.

You can choose any recipe for each meal without blowing your calorie count. Try as many recipes as possible so your taste buds don't get bored. You're bound to have a few favorites that you choose to eat more often. And of course you have more options. You can check for tons of additional recipes on our www.thinin10.com website or from another sensible weight-loss plan such as Weight Watchers or the Dash Diet.

You can use the recipes in each chapter to help create your menu for the week and then make your shopping list and stock your fridge. That's it. It really is that simple. We've limited the ingredients list to basic items that most people are likely to have on hand. This keeps shopping to a minimum.

Liquid Sabotage

Don't forget that beverages contain calories too. One 12-ounce cola or beer contains about 140 calories. That's more than two-thirds of your discretionary calories for the day. If you choose to drink soda or alcohol, be aware that this means giving up something else to commit to the plan. In the evening, you can choose to indulge in a wine spritzer, but at 100 calories, that's half your daily discretionary calories.

For the most part, we recommend avoiding calories in liquid form. They tend not to be very filling and don't do much to satisfy your hunger. On the flip side, some studies indicate that drinking water or no-calorie seltzer can help you feel full and eat less. Plus, you can drink as much of it as you want without damaging your waistline.

To Veg or Not to Veg

Lauren O'Connor, a registered dietitian and owner of Nutri-Savvy in Los Angeles, is often asked: Which is better for me? The fake meat found in veggie burgers or real lean meat?

While swapping out real meat for faux meat may sound like a healthy move, it may not be. It's true that veggie "meat" sometimes contains less saturated fat and more protein than the real deal, but there are other things to consider. Besides being highly processed, the soy protein found in products where veggies masquerade as meat is not as high quality as natural soy sources such as tofu or edamame. Additionally, alternative protein patties tend to contain mountains of salt and other forms of hidden sodium, including monosodium glutamate (MSG) and soy sauce. They're sometimes loaded with added sugars in the form of dextrose and maltodextrin too. Additionally, the hydrolyzed vegetable proteins found in these products have been known to break down into glutamate, a substance that may combine with sodium to form MSG and other not-so-healthy chemicals.

If you do decide to buy these products, check the ingredient list— if a product lists chemical names that require three years of Latin to pronounce, it's not a healthy purchase. You're better off eating fresh or frozen veggies and eating legumes for protein.

Diet soda drinkers seem to have the most trouble making the switch to water. Part of this is psychological. Why kick a diet soda habit when it has no calories and so cannot contribute to weight gain? As previously mentioned, some preliminary evidence suggests that drinking diet soda is actually connected with weight gain. If nothing else, diet soda contains chemicals that don't benefit your body in any way. As we wait for better scientific studies on diet soda, we suggest kicking the diet soda habit and drinking plain water—zest it up with a slice of lemon or lime.

CHAPTER

9 | Breakfast in 10
Minutes or Less

"I can't usually stomach eating breakfast first thing in the morning, but the smoothie recipe was perfect for my busy schedule and minimal appetite."
—Molly, original *Thin in 10* focus group member

Skipping breakfast is a weight-loss strategy that's bound to backfire. Although breakfast skippers figure they're saving calories, they tend to eat more calories overall. Most people who skip breakfast have worse eating behaviors and exercise less than breakfast eaters, and as a result they typically weigh more and have thicker waists. They're also more susceptible to a range of health problems, including high cholesterol and elevated insulin levels, both of which are linked to continued increases in body size.

Study after study finds that breakfast skippers are the least successful at losing weight, in both the short and the long term. On the flip side, the National Weight Control Registry, an ongoing project that examines weight-loss strategies that work, reports that 80 percent of people who maintain weight loss for extended periods of time commit to eating breakfast every single day. This doesn't mean eating breakfast is the cause of weight loss, but it is certainly an established habit many successful losers swear by.

While regular breakfast eating is consistently and reliably associated with healthy weight, it's important to understand that there is nothing magical about consuming calories in the morning. They aren't inherently special or different than afternoon and nighttime calories. Rather, it's simply that passing up the morning meal wreaks havoc on eating habits, blood sugar, metabolism, and willpower, compelling you to act on the urges to overeat later in the day. Forgoing the first meal of the day essentially tricks the brain into thinking you want higher-calorie foods that fatten you up, or at least increases your risk for weight gain. This is why we're so adamant that breakfast be a part of your *Thin in 10* makeover.

Thin in 10 in the A.M.

A good breakfast should be about 300 calories, which is roughly what our breakfast recipes and recommendations contain. Fewer calories, and the meal won't carry you through the morning without a blood sugar crash before your snack or lunchtime. More calories, and you defeat the purpose of eating this meal—research shows that consuming a high-fat, high-calorie breakfast is no more effective for beating later-in-the-day cravings or consuming fewer overall calories than eating a lighter, healthier morning meal.

Although you want a good balance of fat and carbs for energy and protein for staying power, we prefer not to think about food entirely in terms of its components. You should eat something that makes you happy yet still keeps you healthy. The breakfast recipes in this chapter fit the bill. They're packed with nutrition, plus there's something tasty here for everyone from egg lovers to carb cravers.

"You should eat something that makes you happy yet still keeps you healthy."

We strongly advise you to take the few minutes needed to whip up these recipes at home rather than hitting the drive-through or the deli on your way to work. This will help you keep the calories as well as the sugar, sodium, and all the other bad stuff under control—something that's almost impossible to do when your breakfast comes wrapped in plastic. None of the recipes takes more than 10 minutes to make, so no excuses. More quick, easy, and delicious breakfast options are available at www.thinin10.com.

Breakfast Takeaways

- Cook and eat breakfast at home at least six days a week.
- The only kitchen tools required for these meals are a microwave, baking sheet, nonstick skillet, and a good spatula. Oh, and a toaster and stove too!
- Each recipe serves one and takes 10 minutes or less from start to finish (cleanup is pretty quick too).

The *Thin in 10* Breakfast Recipes (300 calories)

Apple Spice Oatmeal

This delicious dish is packed with vitamin C and heart-healthy B vitamins. It satisfies your sweet tooth without adding any sugar, honey, agave, brown rice syrup, or sugar substitute.

Ingredients

1/2 cup dried oats

2 tbsp raisins

3 tbsp applesauce, unsweetened

1 tbsp sliced almonds (or toasted pumpkin seeds or nuts/seeds of your choice)

1 tsp cinnamon

1/4 cup 1% milk

1 cup water

Directions

1. Boil the water.
2. Add oats and raisins. Heat until most of the water is absorbed.
3. Add applesauce and almonds.
4. Cover for 1–3 minutes, or until all of the water is absorbed.
5. Add cinnamon and milk.

Nutrition Facts

Cal 300, Fat 7 grams (g), Fiber 8 g, Sugar 23 g, Protein 9 g, Sodium 340 milligram (mg)

Cinnamon Bagel with Blueberry Cream Cheese

You don't have to give up your morning bagel for weight loss; just give it a flavorful makeover to keep it waistline friendly! Feel free to swap out the blueberries and replace with your favorite berry instead.

Ingredients

1 mini cinnamon raisin bagel (your favorite mini or 100–110 calorie bagel thin)

2 tbsp low-fat whipped cream cheese

1/2 cup blueberries, fresh or frozen

2 tangerines

1 tbsp walnuts

Directions

1. Slice bagel in half, and toast if desired.
2. Mix thawed blueberries into whipped cream cheese (you may choose to add fewer blueberries to the cream cheese, and serve the remainder on the side)
3. Spread the blueberry cream cheese onto each bagel half.
4. Serve with tangerines and walnuts (if you'd like a little crunch, add them into your "bagel sandwich").

Nutrition Facts

Cal 270, Fat 9 g, Fiber 6 g, Sugar 25 g, Protein 7 g, Sodium 180 mg

RD Recommendation: Labels

Lauren says: Always read your labels. Bagels vary in calories (as well as sodium content), whether large or small. Some mini bagels may be 120 calories while others are 70. Most bagel thins are between 110 and 120 calories. Opt for lower sodium as much as possible. Try to limit the sodium to 300 mg or less per serving

Apple 'jacks with Peanut Butter

Pancakes? Yes, please! Eating these yummy protein-rich pancakes prevent you from having a sugar crash later. If you prefer yours sweeter, add one-third of a banana and use 2 teaspoons of peanut butter instead of 1 tablespoon. Then mash the banana and remaining peanut butter together to use as your spread. Bonus: This reduces the fat!

Ingredients

2 4" frozen pancakes (our dietitian recommends multigrain— 60 calories each)

1 tbsp peanut butter

1/2 cup chunky, unsweetened applesauce (or smooth)

1 tsp cinnamon

2 thin slices of a medium apple (for garnish)

Directions

1. Heat pancakes according to package instructions (toaster oven or microwave).
2. Spread peanut butter between the two pancakes.
3. Heat applesauce on the stove or in the microwave.
4. Top your pancake sandwich with applesauce and garnish with apple slices and cinnamon.

Nutrition Facts

Cal 300, Fat 11 g, Fiber 5 g, Sugar 16 g, Protein 6 g, Sodium 650 mg

RD Recommendation: Peanut Butter

Peanut butter should be made with just peanuts and a little salt. Look for natural versions with no added sugars, hydrogenated oils, or any other additives. And if you're allergic to peanuts, use a suitable substitution.

Choco-Banana Smoothie

This low-sodium liquid breakfast is a great source of potassium and magnesium. Plus, it has enough protein to keep the munchies at bay. (Jessica loves it because it has chocolate in it!)

Ingredients

1 cup 1% milk

1 medium banana

1 tbsp unsweetened cocoa powder

10 almonds

Directions

1. Slice the banana into small disks for easier blending and pureé all ingredients in a blender.
2. Pour into serving cup and enjoy!

Nutrition Facts

Cal 300, Fat 9 g, Fiber 6 g, Sugar 32 g, Protein 14 g, Sodium 130 mg

Eggs Benedict Light

This is a light and easy makeover of a classic breakfast. It makes the perfect breakfast indulgence!

Ingredients

1 large egg

2 tbsp Greek nonfat yogurt (or 1/2 tbsp reduced-fat mayonnaise)

1 tsp light butter spread

1/2 tsp (or to taste) lemon juice

1 multigrain English muffin (100 calorie) or bagel thin lightly toasted (not crunchy)

1 apple

Directions

1. Poach the egg (or scramble it with nonstick spray). (Instead of using the stove, try poaching an egg in the microwave by filling a 1-cup microwaveable bowl or cup with 1/2 cup water, gently crack in egg, add a tiny drop of vinegar, and microwave covered for about 1 minute.)
2. Toast the English muffin.
3. Mix yogurt (or mayo) with juice and cooled, melted butter spread.

continued

4. Place egg on top of the English muffin and garnish with lemon yogurt mixture.
5. Cut apple into slices and enjoy on the side, along with the other half of the muffin (or save for later).

Nutrition Facts

Cal 280, Fat 6 g, Fiber 13 g, Sugar 22 g, Protein 14 g, Sodium 320 mg

Scrambled Eggs with Toast

Start your day off with broccoli, a nutrient-dense veggie full of vitamins C, K, A, and folate. Broccoli is a good source of dietary fiber and calcium. If you just can't stomach it this early in the morning, substitute another veggie of your choice.

Ingredients

2 eggs
1/2 cup broccoli crowns, fresh or frozen thawed (chop into bits or use small broccoli crowns)
1 tsp olive oil

1 piece multigrain toast (our dietitian recommends Orowheat Double Fiber—70 calories per slice or any 80-calorie wholegrain bread)
1 tbsp regular cream cheese

Directions

1. Scramble the eggs and broccoli together in a pan lightly coated with olive oil.
2. Toast bread and spread with cream cheese.

Nutrition Facts

Cal 300, Fat 16 g, Fiber 7 g, Sugar 5 g, Protein 19 g, Sodium 350 mg

RD Recommendation: Cereal

A serving of cereal and milk for breakfast meets our calorie recommendations. However, don't be fooled by the claims listed on cereal boxes—so many cereals labeled as "healthy" really aren't. Check the nutrition labels; look for cereals with at least 3 g of fiber and no more than 12 g of sugar.

RD Recommendation: Bread

Any type of bread you buy, whether it's sandwich bread, sandwich thins, or tortillas, should be whole grain and 100 percent whole wheat (if you're not gluten intolerant). Be sure to check the ingredient list for sugars and other additives (some reduced-calorie breads add sugar or sweeteners to make up for flavor lost with calories). High-fiber varieties (3 g of fiber or more per serving) are popping up in most major super-markets, some with as much as 14 g of fiber per serving. These are good choices because fiber helps you feel full, maintains regularity, and helps maintain healthy cholesterol levels.

If You Must . . .

Starbucks New York Everything Bagel

A New York–style bagel topped with Asiago cheese, poppy and sesame seeds, onion, and garlic.

Cal 280, Fat 2 g, Fiber 2 g, Sugar 5 g, Protein 10 g, Sodium 500 mg
Top it with 1 tbsp cream cheese to add 51 cal, 5 g fat, 43 mg sodium, 1 g protein.

Dunkin Donuts Egg on English Muffin

English muffin, egg patty, and cheese.

Cal 320, Fat 15g, Fiber 1 g, Sugar 3 g, Protein 14 g, Sodium 820 mg
Note how high that sodium count is! While this breakfast would sat-isfy your calorie goal, it is a killer on your sodium intake—and this is only breakfast!

CHAPTER 10 | Lunch in 10 Minutes or Less

"The lunches are so easy to fix, they're a no-brainer. And I have really learned how to be mindful about eating and can gauge portion sizes now—I can see my waist! I'm in shock!"
—Sharon, original *Thin in 10* focus group member

You're less likely to skip lunch than breakfast, but if you're not careful it's the meal that can easily sabotage your efforts. The two biggest mistakes we see people make with lunch are skimping on calories so their hunger becomes out of control later in the day or losing control of calories by dining out too often.

The first problem creates issues similar to skipping breakfast. Any time you skip or skimp on a meal, you set yourself up for disaster down the road. Going all the way from the morning into the evening without sufficiently refueling your body's energy supply makes you vulnerable to bad choices. Your blood sugar crashes, making it harder to concentrate or be productive. Your mood takes a nosedive. You can't get motivated to work out. Pretty soon all you want to do is hit the vending machine, bakery, or drive-through. Any calories you "saved" by cutting way back on calories earlier in the day is more than made up for with an evening binge.

The second problem can be a bit tougher to overcome. Not too many people brown-bag, or prepare their own lunch, anymore. Lunch is the meal most frequently purchased away from home. According to the National Restaurant Association, nearly 61 percent of people buy rather than make their lunch each day, with an average cost of nearly $10. So making your own lunch not only helps control your calories but cushions your budget too.

We do understand that it might be a big adjustment to make your own lunch, especially during the week and especially if you're a student or busy parent, or if you work outside the home. But if you're serious about transforming your body, this change is necessary. It would be a shame to get most of the plan right but then not achieve the results you want because you blew something as simple as lunch. The good news? We're bringing the brown-bag lunch back—and you don't have to worry about putting too much effort into it.

> "Lunch is the meal most frequently purchased away from home."

We've made it ridiculously easy to get with the program. This chapter includes eight choices for delicious do-it-yourself lunches that total about 400 calories each. That's enough fuel to keep you satisfied until a later snack or dinner but not so much that you need to cut back elsewhere. As with all of our recipes, each lunch takes less than 10 minutes to make from the moment you gather the ingredients to the moment you place the food in your lunch bag. Even for those of us who don't love to cook, that's doable.

Lunch Takeaways

- Prepare and eat your own lunch at least six days a week.
- Most of these recipes don't require cooking, but one requires a non-stick skillet and a good spatula. You'll need a toaster, oh, and a stove too!
- Each recipe serves one and takes 10 minutes (many much less) from start to finish (cleanup is pretty quick too).

The *Thin in 10* Lunch Recipes (400 calories)

Peanut Butter & Jelly Roll with Banana

You are never too old to enjoy this classic brown-bag favorite. It's also a great energy-boosting meal that keeps you satisfied through the afternoon slump.

Ingredients

1 100–120 calorie tortilla (our dietitian recommends an Old El Paso 8", Grandma's 6", or La Tortilla Smart & Delicious, which has a variety of healthy whole-grain ingredients and 12 g dietary fiber)

1 tbsp peanut butter

1 tbsp strawberry jam

1 medium banana

Directions

1. Spread peanut butter and jam onto the tortilla.
2. Roll up and slice in half, or enjoy the roll-up in bite-size 1/2" pieces.
3. Serve with a medium banana.

Nutrition Facts

Cal 360, Fat 11 g, Fiber 5 g, Sugar 32 g, Protein 7 g, Sodium 280 mg

Cucumber Yogurt Salad in a Pita

This easy-to-eat pita includes several servings of fruits and vegetables—which are weight-loss friendly and fiber rich.

Ingredients

1/2 cucumber, peeled, quartered lengthwise, and sliced into chunks

1/4 cup nonfat Greek yogurt

1/4 tsp dried dill (or 1 tsp fresh dill)

2 oz precooked chicken strips (our dietitian likes Applegate Naturals brand or Hormel Natural Choice)

1 romaine lettuce leaf

1 6½" pita (about 160 cal, equivalent to 2 slices of bread)

1 small apple

10–14 baby carrots (1/2 cup)

Salt or no-salt seasoning (to taste)

continued

Directions

1. Gently mix the cucumber chunks, yogurt, and dill.
2. Sprinkle on salt (or a no-salt vegetable seasoning) to taste.
3. Add chicken strips.
4. Cut the pita in half and place one half inside the other (this holds the ingredients better than just one).
5. Place the lettuce leaf in the pita and then scoop in the cucumber salad mixture.
6. Enjoy with the apple and some baby carrots.

Nutrition Facts

Cal 400, Fat 2½ g, Fiber 11 g, Sugar 25 g, Protein 30 g, Sodium 590 mg

Turkey with Provolone & Basil Roll-Up

This is a dressed-up version of a classic turkey sandwich. Although the name sounds fancy, it's simple to make!

Ingredients

2 oz deli turkey, thinly sliced
1 oz provolone cheese
1 flour tortilla (8")
1 tbsp fat-free Greek yogurt (or light mayonnaise, or 1/2 tbsp of each)

6 large or 12 small fresh basil leaves
1/2 cup mixed salad greens
2–4 slices cucumber (sliced lengthwise to fit into roll)
1 medium pear

Directions

1. Spread yogurt or light mayo on the tortilla.
2. Layer with turkey, cheese, basil, cucumber, and salad greens.
3. Roll up and enjoy with a pear.

Nutrition Facts

Cal 390, Fat 10 g, Fiber 7 g, Sugar 21 g, Protein 26 g, Sodium 640 mg

Curried "Tuna" Salad

Like tuna salad? You'll love this exotic twist on the traditional tuna salad sandwich.
Not a fan of salmon? No problem. It is just as delish with regular tuna fish.

Ingredients

3 oz unsalted canned salmon (or
   tuna fish), drained and flaked
1 tbsp light mayo
1/2 cup chopped celery
1 tbsp cranberries
1 tbsp chopped walnuts
1 tsp yellow curry powder

1 piece multigrain toast (our
   dietitian likes Sara Lee Delightful
   Wheat Bakery bread—45 cal per
   slice, or Orowheat Double Fiber,
   70 cal per slice)
2 romaine lettuce leaves

Directions

1. In a bowl, mix all ingredients together except the bread and lettuce.
2. Spread mixture onto one piece of toast; then top with lettuce and
   other piece of toast (or serve open faced).

Nutrition Facts

Cal 400, Fat 17 g, Fiber 5 g, Sugar 15 g, Protein 24 g, Sodium 410 mg

RD Recommendation: Mayo

When purchasing mayonnaise, look for a short list of simple, natural
ingredients such as eggs, olive oil, vinegar, mustard, and lemon juice.
Avoid any product with a laundry list of chemicals. Tip: 1/2 tablespoon
of mayo is about 45 calories. Two tablespoons of nonfat yogurt have
only 15–18 calories. You can substitute yogurt for mayonnaise in most
recipes or use reduced-fat mayonnaise if you prefer the taste.

'Tatta in a Pocket

Eggs are a great source of protein—plus, they've been proven to aid in weight loss, yay!—and they are perfect at any meal. We love eating eggs for lunch with this recipe.

Ingredients

1 egg

1/4 cup fajita-style vegetables (bell peppers and onions), fresh or frozen and thawed

Nonstick cooking spray

1 slice deli ham, thinly sliced

1/2 tbsp Parmesan cheese, grated

1 tbsp 1% milk

1 tbsp water

1/2 cup fresh baby spinach

1/2 whole-wheat pita

1 tsp pesto sauce

Tomato

1 medium apple

Directions

1. Whisk egg with milk in a bowl.
2. Sauté onions and peppers over medium heat in a pan coated with cooking spray. Cook until soft. Add water as needed to keep vegetables from sticking to pan.
3. Pour in egg and milk mixture, cheese, and ham. Cook until done in the center.
4. Spread pesto inside the pita. Using a spatula, loosen egg mixture on the edges of the pan and fold into pita with spinach and a couple slices of tomato. Serve with an apple.

Nutrition Facts

Cal 390, Fat 13 g, Fiber 9 g, Sugar 26 g, Protein 20 g, Sodium 410 mg

Pear & Brie Melt

This delicious melt-in-your mouth lunch is an easy treat that only feels indulgent.

Ingredients

2 slices hearty whole-wheat bread (we like Pepperidge Farm 100 percent whole wheat, stone ground—90 calories per slice)

1 oz (2 tbsp) brie spread

1 medium pear, sliced

1/2 cup baby carrots

continued

Directions

1. Spread brie onto slices of bread.
2. Top one slice with thin slices of pear.
3. Place other piece of bread on top.
4. Place in toaster oven until desired doneness.
5. Serve with side of baby carrots.

Nutrition Facts

Cal 400, Fat 9 g, Fiber 11 g, Sugars 27 g, Protein 13 g, Sodium 550 mg

Crunchy Strawberry Cream Cheese Muffin

This sandwich has everything—a nice blend of sweet, crunchy, and creamy. It's full of protein and fiber to help hold you over until dinner.

Ingredients

1 whole-wheat English muffin
1 oz (2 tbsp) whipped cream cheese
1/4 cup sliced strawberries (3–4 medium berries)
1 tbsp chopped walnuts
1 medium apple

Directions

1. Toast the English muffin.
2. Spread on cream cheese and add sliced strawberries and walnuts evenly on the two muffin halves.
3. Enjoy with a crisp, delicious apple.

Nutrition Facts

Cal 350, Fat 13 g, Fiber 10 g, Sugar 28 g, Protein 9 g, Sodium 310 mg

RD Recommendation: Canned Salmon or Tuna

When scanning the shelves for salmon or tuna, look for the lowest amounts of potentially harmful mercury. Choose light tuna that's water-packed to save on calories. Canned wild salmon is one of your best sources for omega-3s.

Cucumber Salmon Flatbread Roll

If you are a fan of sushi, this is a great alternative to the seaweed way and labor-intensive rolling.

Ingredients

1 flour tortilla (we recommend La Tortilla Factory Smart & Delicious 100-calorie tortillas or Garden of Eatin' from Hain Celestial Group)

1 oz (2 tbsp) whipped cream cheese
1 oz lox (smoked salmon)
1 cucumber, sliced thinly lengthwise
1 medium pear

Directions

1. Spread lox and cream cheese onto the tortilla, add cucumber slices; then roll and enjoy!
2. Eat with a refreshing pear.

Nutrition Facts

Cal 390, Fat 11 g, Fiber 11 g, Sugar 25 g, Protein 14 g, Sodium 800 mg

If You Must . . .

KFC Snacker with Crispy Strip

Without sauce
Cal 260, Fat 9 g, Fiber 2 g, Sugar 4 g, Protein 15 g, Sodium 550 mg

With green beans
Cal 25, Fat 0 g, Fiber 2 g, Sugar 1g, Protein 1 g, Sodium 260 mg

With corn on cob (3")
Cal 70, Fat 1/2 g, Fiber 2 g, Sugar 3 g, Protein 2 g, Sodium 0 mg

Taco Bell Chicken Fresco Crunchy Tacos

With salsa, lettuce, seasoned chicken, taco shell
Cal 290, Fat 15 g, Fiber 3 g, Sugar 1 g, Protein 6 g, Sodium 620 mg

continued

If You Must...

Subway Fresh Fit Choices

Black Forest ham sandwich (6")
Cal 290, Fat 6 g, Fiber 5 g, Sugar 8 g, Protein 18 g, Sodium 830 mg

Oven-roasted chicken sandwich (6")
Cal 320, Fat 5 g, Fiber 5 g, Sugar 8 g, Protein 23 g, Sodium 640 mg

Lauren says, "Yikes!" Most of these choices are high in sodium. This is just another reminder to make eating out a rare occurrence, though we grudgingly admit all of these selections would fit into your calorie budget.

CHAPTER 11

Dinner in 10 Minutes or Less

"I am more aware of what I eat, and this meal plan is easy to adapt to and so simple to follow."
—Christina, original *Thin in 10* focus group member

Ah, dinner. While it's a great idea in theory to cook yourself a wholesome, nutritious evening meal that won't sabotage your diet, how often do you actually pull that off? By the time the thought of making dinner pops into your head, you're probably too hungry or tired, or you have nothing in the pantry. Even for people who love to cook, there are times when takeout sounds so much easier.

We know that for many people, dinner is the most challenging meal to make at home—but for the sake of your entire family's waistline (and wallet), we're going to ask you to eat in. The recipes in this chapter make it easy to whip up a healthy, satisfying meal for yourself or your entire family, all in less time than it takes to pick up takeout. Every one of these family-friendly meals can go from your pantry to the table in 10 minutes (or less). And did we mention they are delicious? We have included a variety of dinner options, knowing that we don't all like the same things. Some might not like fish or red meat. Others are fans of meat and potatoes and want something hearty for dinner each night. We've got it. All of our dinner recipes come in at about 600 calories, which should be plenty satisfying and prevent midnight snack runs.

If you have special dietary considerations, make substitutions in the recipes as you see fit or visit our website at www.thinin10.com for additional, specialty recipe options.

Dinner Takeaways

- Cook and eat dinner at home at least six days a week.
- The only cooking tools needed for these recipes are a microwave, a baking sheet, a nonstick skillet, and a good spatula. Oh, and a stove too!
- Each recipe serves one and takes 10 minutes or less from start to finish (cleanup is pretty quick too).

The *Thin in 10* Dinner Recipes (600 calories)

Sloppy Jo'sephines and Carrot-Raisin Slaw

Try this delicious twist on Sloppy Joes that swaps out ground beef for lean chicken strips and serve it up with a side of carrot-raisin slaw for a satisfying, hearty meal sans extra fat. Who says this has to be a "man's meal"?

Ingredients for the Sloppy Jo'sephines

1 whole-wheat hamburger bun
3 oz low-sodium chicken strips (our dietitian likes Applegate brand)
3 tbsp low-sodium BBQ sauce (our dietitian prefers Bob Evans, a low-sodium brand)
1/2 cup bell peppers and onions, fresh or frozen and thawed

Ingredients for the Slaw

1/2 cup grated carrots (look for pregrated carrots for easier prep)
1/4 cup nonfat Greek yogurt
2 tbsp raisins
1/4 tsp cinnamon
1/2 cup sliced apples
1 tsp honey

continued

Directions

1. For the Sloppy Jo'sephine, toast the bun for 2–4 minutes until desired crispness.
2. Heat BBQ sauce mixed with chicken and thawed veggies on stove over low-medium heat until warm.
3. For the carrot-raisin slaw, mix grated carrots, sliced apple, cinnamon, raisins, honey, and Greek yogurt.
4. Place chicken and veggie mixture on bun and serve with the slaw.

Nutrition Facts

Cal 560, Fat 3½ g, Fiber 12 g, Sugar 51 g, Protein 40 g, Sodium 740 mg

Parmesan-Crusted Chicken Bake with Mashed Potatoes and Apple Salad

This is so good, it satisfies cravings for fried chicken. The mashed potatoes are decadently creamy but still "light." And the crunchy apple salad is a great way to complete the meal.

Ingredients for the Chicken

1/4 cup bread crumbs (such as Panko)

4 oz skinless, boneless chicken breast, pounded and cut into 4 pieces

1 egg white

2 tbsp flour

2 tbsp Parmesan cheese (preferably reduced fat), grated

1/2 tsp Italian seasoning (no salt added)

1/2 tsp minced garlic (dried)

2 tbsp nonfat Greek yogurt

2 tsp honey Dijon mustard (look for brands with limited ingredients, mainly mustard and honey)

Nonstick cooking spray or 2 tsp olive oil

Ingredients for the Mashed Potatoes

1/2 cup broccoli

1/3 cup mashed potato flakes (if you prefer mashed potatoes from scratch, by all means go ahead and make them—we kept them instant to save you some time. RD Lauren

approves this shortcut.)

1 tsp light butter spread (such as Smart Balance Light)

1/3 cup water

2 tbsp 1% milk

continued

Ingredients for the Apple Salad

1 cup butter lettuce or lettuce of
   choice, chopped
1 medium apple, thinly sliced

1 tbsp crumbled blue cheese
1 tbsp low-sodium balsamic
   vinaigrette

Directions for the Chicken

1. Set a kettle or pot of water to boil.
2. Whisk egg white in a bowl and prepare a plate with the flour for dipping.
3. In a small bowl, mix yogurt and honey Dijon mustard. Set aside.
4. In a separate bowl, mix bread crumbs, Parmesan, garlic, and Italian seasoning.
7. Heat pan over low heat.
8. Dip each chicken piece into flour, then egg white, and finally roll into bread-crumb mixture.
9. Add coated chicken to hot pan.
10. Heat about 2–3 minutes each side until golden brown (chicken should no longer be pink inside; test doneness by cutting with a knife or fork).

Directions for the Potatoes

1. Place broccoli in a microwave-safe bowl with a little water and cover with a plate; microwave for about 3 minutes.
2. Add boiling water to potato flakes and prepare according to package instructions (adding in milk, water, and light butter).
3. Mix in steamed broccoli and light butter.

Directions for the Apple Salad

1. Mix blue cheese and balsamic vinaigrette dressing with lettuce and apples.

Nutrition Facts

Cal 590, Fat 15 g, Fiber 9 g, Sugar 33 g, Protein 40 g, Sodium 730 mg

Chili Lime Chicken Fajitas with Rice and Avocado Salad

One of Liz's favorites! This recipe is easy to make, tasty, and satisfying (a hit for the whole family).

Ingredients for the Fajitas

2 oz cooked chicken strips (our dietitian likes Applegate Organics, with less than 300 mg of sodium per serving)

1 cup fajita-style vegetables (bell peppers and onions), fresh or frozen and thawed

1/4 tsp chili powder or chili flakes

2 tbsp water

1 tsp olive oil

1 tbsp lime juice—or squeeze whole lime

1/2 cup sliced zucchini

1 6" flour tortilla

1/2 cup diced tomatoes

1/2 cup microwavable rice

Ingredients for the Salad

1 cup mixed greens

1/5 medium avocado

1 tbsp toasted pumpkin seeds, unsalted

1 tsp olive oil

Juice of 1 lime

Directions

1. Heat oil in a pan; then add vegetables and seasonings.
2. Add water as necessary so vegetables don't stick to pan.
3. Prepare rice according to directions.
4. When vegetables are soft, add chicken to pan and heat until warm.
5. Toss all salad ingredients together.
6. Serve fajita mix-ins (chicken and seasoned vegetables) over flour tortilla with a side of rice and salad.

Nutrition Facts

Cal 560, Fat 21 g, Fiber 10 g, Sugar 19 g, Protein 29 g, Sodium 640 mg

Meat 'n' Potatoes Stew and Tossed Salad

So hardy and satisfying, this recipe often becomes a go-to comfort food. The salad adds a pop of fresh greens to the meal.

Ingredients for the Stew

1/2 can beef and vegetables soup (we like Campbell's Select Harvest Vegetable Beef and Barley)

1 medium boiled potato (or 2/3 cup potato flakes for mashed potato)

1/2 cup canned garbanzo beans, drained

1/4 tsp minced garlic, dried

3 oz fresh, ground hamburger, 90% lean

Ingredients for the Salad

1 cup fresh baby spinach

1 tsp olive oil

1/2 tsp balsamic vinegar

Directions

1. Heat soup on stove over low heat.
2. In another pot, prepare potato (or potato flakes).
3. While potato is cooking and soup is heating, heat garlic, garbanzo beans, and ground hamburger in non-stick pan over medium heat for 3–5 minutes (make sure meat is fully cooked).
4. Mix all together in a bowl.
5. Serve with tossed salad made of spinach leaves, olive oil, and balsamic vinegar.

Nutrition Facts

Cal. 540, Fat 15 g, Fiber 11 g, Sugar 9 g, Protein 36 g, Sodium 610 mg

RD Recommendation: Oil

Olive oil is often touted for its omega-3 fatty acids, but it's really the monounsaturated fats that make it a superstar. Choose extra-virgin, cold-pressed to ensure you are getting the heart-healthy monounsaturated fats and antioxidant omega-3s. Use in moderation to keep saturated fats within recommended daily intake, which the American Heart Association advises should be limited to less than 7 percent of daily intake.

Beef & Bean Chili with Corn

We love the rich flavor of this dish. It tastes like a chili that's simmered in the pot for hours, but it's only 10 minutes from pan to plate!

Ingredients

4 oz lean ground beef

1/8 tsp minced garlic, dried

1/2 cup low-sodium marinara sauce

1/2 cup fresh or canned mushrooms, sliced (rinse and drain if using canned)

1 tbsp thick and chunky salsa (hot or medium)

1/2 cup canned kidney beans, drained

1/2 tsp Worcestershire sauce

1/2 cup bell peppers and onions, fresh or frozen and thawed

1 cup frozen corn kernels, thawed and divided

1/2 pita

Nonstick cooking spray

Directions

1. Spray nonstick cooking oil in pan over low-medium heat.
2. Cook ground beef until browned thoroughly, breaking it up as you go.
3. Stir in marinara sauce, garlic, sliced mushrooms, kidney beans, 1/2 cup corn, Worcestershire sauce, bell peppers and onions, and salsa.
4. Heat until warmed.
5. Serve with pita and remaining 1/2 cup of corn.

Nutrition Facts

Cal 560, Fat 9 g, Fiber 16 g, Sugar 29 g, Protein 42 g, Sodium 750 mg

RD Recommendation: Canned Beans

Look for "low-sodium," "50% less sodium" or "no-salt added" on the label, and no more than 300 mg of sodium per serving. The richer the color, the higher the nutrient content, so choose red kidney, pinto, and black beans for antioxidants.

Zesty Pasta with Sausage & Peppers

Got a craving for Italian? This light version of a traditional pasta dish is just the ticket! If you're not an almond fan, leave them out and save a few calories.

Ingredients

2 oz uncooked penne pasta
1/2 chicken apple sausage, sliced
   (our dietitian recommends
   a brand with no nitrates)
1/2 cup onions and bell peppers,
   fresh or frozen and thawed
1/2 tsp Worcestershire sauce
1/8 tsp minced garlic, dried

1/2 cup low-sodium marinara
   sauce
1/8 tsp no-salt veggie seasoning
2 oz fresh or canned mushrooms,
   sliced (if using canned, rinse and
   drain)
2 tbsp Parmesan cheese, grated
1/2 cup frozen green beans, thawed
1 tbsp sliced almonds

Directions

1. Boil water and cook pasta according to package instructions.
2. In a pan over medium heat, add sausage pieces, onions and peppers, Worcestershire sauce, marinara sauce, mushrooms, and spices.
3. Heat until warm.
4. Drain pasta and add to sauce.
5. Top with Parmesan cheese.
6. Serve with green beans (microwave 1–2 minutes or cook over the stove).
7. Garnish beans with sliced almonds.

Nutrition Facts

Cal 520, Fat 16g, Fiber 7g, Sugar 17g, Protein 25g, Sodium 690 mg

RD Recommendation: Chicken Broth

Low-sodium or unsalted is your best bet when purchasing chicken broth since regular versions may contain nearly 900 mg of sodium per cup. Opt for organic when possible. To save calories, use chicken broth or water instead of extra oil to keep meats or veggies from sticking to a skillet during meal prep.

Shepherd's Pie

Did you ever think you'd be able to eat something so indulgent on any weight-loss plan?

Ingredients

2/3 cup potato flakes

1/4 cup 1% milk (or milk substitute such as soy or almond milk)

2/3 cup water (for potatoes) plus 1/4 cup water (for vegetables; or use 1/4 cup chicken broth)

1 tbsp light butter spread (such as Smart Balance Light)

1 cup frozen mixed vegetables, thawed

1/2 cup frozen chopped spinach, thawed

2 tbsp chopped green onions (about two strands)

4 oz lean ground beef

2 tbsp bread crumbs (such as Panko)

1 tsp olive oil

2 tsp Italian seasoning herbs (no salt added)

1 tbsp flour

Nonstick cooking spray

Directions

1. Put 2 cups of water in a pot to boil or use a kettle.
2. Heat olive oil in a pan over medium heat; then add green onions and sauté for about 2 minutes.
3. Add ground beef and Italian seasoning to pan, and stir until all sides are completely browned.
4. Mix in vegetable blend and spinach.
5. Add 1/4 cup water (or chicken broth) and mix in flour, heating until thickened.
6. In a bowl, mix potato flakes with 2/3 cup water, milk, and 2 tsp of light butter until the mashed potatoes become thick and fluffy.
7. Place 2 tbsp of mashed potatoes in two sections of the muffin tin sprayed with nonstick oil. Divide the vegetables and meat mixture evenly between the two so it reaches the top of the rim (don't worry if there are excess vegetables—you can serve those on the side).
8. Top with remaining mashed potatoes.
9. Sprinkle with Panko bread crumbs and dot the tops of each pie with the remaining light butter.
10. Place under broiler for 1–3 minutes until just browned.

Nutrition Facts

Cal 570, Fat 15 g, Fiber 8 g, Sugar 12 g, Protein 35 g, Sodium 450 mg

Shrimp Nonfried Rice

If you're used to reaching for the Chinese takeout menu, this recipe should satisfy that craving. It's a lighter, much healthier version of a takeout classic—and it's so tasty you won't even miss the fat and calories!

Ingredients

1/2 cup microwavable brown rice

1 tsp olive oil

2 tbsp scallions, chopped

2 tbsp chopped walnuts

1 tsp light butter spread (we recommend Smart Balance Light)

1 tsp soy sauce

1 tbsp raisins

1/2 cup frozen peas, carrots, and corn blend, thawed (no sodium, no sauce, no seasoning added)

3 oz cooked shrimp

1 cup fresh baby spinach

Directions

1. Wash and cook the rice according to package instructions.
2. In a separate pan, sauté the scallions with the walnuts and raisins in olive oil over medium heat until the scallions are soft and the walnuts are toasty (about 3 minutes).
3. When the rice is done, add butter, and then mix in the scallions, walnuts, raisins, veggies, and shrimp.
4. Simmer over low to medium heat on the stove for 2 minutes or until warmed through.
5. Serve on top of the fresh spinach.

Nutrition Facts

Cal 600, Fat 14 g, Sodium 770 mg, Fiber 11 g, Sugar 11 g, Protein 36 g

Shrimp & Avocado Salad

In the mood for a light evening meal? This easy pasta salad makes great use of shrimp and avocado for a delish meal that's perfect for a last-minute dinner.

Ingredients

5 oz cooked shrimp

1/4 medium avocado

3/4 cup diced tomatoes (our dietitian prefers fresh, but look for unsalted if using canned)

Juice of 1 lemon

1 tsp olive oil

2 oz dry rigatoni

1½ cups arugula (or your favorite salad greens)

Pepper to taste

Directions

1. Boil water and cook rigatoni according to package instructions, drain, and cool.
2. Mix remaining ingredients, except arugula, and then toss with the cooked rigatoni.
3. Serve over arugula.

Nutrition Facts

Cal 540, Fat 15 g, Fiber 7 g, Sugar 9 g, Protein 46 g, Sodium 440 mg

Baked Salmon with Lemon Butter, Asparagus and Pasta

Salmon is Jessica's favorite fish and for good reason—it's meaty and flavorful yet low in calories and packed with healthy fats. With the addition of the pasta, this dish has it all!

Ingredients for the Salmon

5 oz salmon fillet (sliced thin)

2 tsp light mayonnaise

2 tsp light butter spread (we recommend Smart Balance Light or other light buttery spread that contains omega-3s)

1 quarter fresh lemon, sliced thin (squeeze the rest in your water for debloating benefits)

15 medium fresh asparagus spears

Nonstick olive oil cooking spray

Pepper to taste

continued

Ingredients for the Pasta

2 oz dry pasta

1/2 cup fresh baby spinach

1 tsp light butter spread

Pepper to taste

Directions

1. Preheat oven to 425 degrees F.
2. Boil 2 cups of water in a saucepan.
3. Rinse and pat salmon dry with paper towel, and then place salmon on a baking sheet sprayed with oil. Cut a few slits in the salmon.
4. Dress salmon with the mayonnaise and insert dots of light butter and lemon into the slits. Bake for about 10 minutes. When water has boiled, add 2 ounces dry pasta, simmering for 7–8 minutes (or according to package instructions; cooking time may vary with pasta used) while salmon is baking.
5. Place the asparagus in a steamer above the pasta's boiling water and cover (about 6 minutes, or until slightly tender but not mushy).
6. Make sure salmon is fully cooked; it should flake easily and no longer be dark pink inside.
7. Set salmon aside and put pasta into serving bowl, mixing in light butter. Gently fold in spinach. Add pepper to taste and squeeze lemon onto the asparagus.

Nutrition Facts

Cal 590, Fat 24 g, Fiber 11 g, Sugar 13 g, Protein 44 g, Sodium 430 mg

Broiled Tilapia with Cheesy Cauliflower & Potatoes

Here's a flavorful recipe for this farm-raised fish that is easy breezy! The creamy, cheesy veggies give it an impressive flavor and texture.

Ingredients

2 tsp light butter spread

1 tsp lemon juice

1/8 tsp salt

1/8 tsp pepper

1/8 tsp dried basil

6 oz tilapia fillet

1 cup frozen cauliflower

1/4 cup shredded cheddar cheese

1/2 cup potatoes, chopped

1 cup butter lettuce

1 sliced tomato

1 tbsp balsamic vinaigrette

continued

Directions

1. Preheat oven to broil.
2. Place chopped potatoes in a microwave-safe dish and microwave on high for 5 minutes. Grease a broiling pan or line the pan with aluminum foil and place tilapia on it.
3. Spread 1 teaspoon light butter over the top of the fillet, and then season with lemon juice, salt, pepper, and basil. Broil a few inches from the heat for 4–5 minutes and then turn the fillet over and repeat.
4. While the fish is broiling, remove potato and mix with 1 teaspoon of butter and set on a serving dish.
5. Place the cauliflower and 2 tablespoons of water in a microwave-safe dish and microwave on high for 4 minutes. Top with shredded cheese and cook for an additional 30 seconds, or until melted.
6. Mix together lettuce, tomato, and vinaigrette in a salad bowl and serve.

Nutrition Facts

Cal 530, Fat 24 g, Fiber 8 g, Sugar 6 g, Protein 50 g, Sodium 460 mg

Fluffy Frittata

This is the ultimate "breakfast for dinner" dish. For variety, lose the ham and swap out the green salad for a fresh fruit salad. Yum! Note: For this recipe, use a frying pan that can be placed in the oven, such as a black cast-iron skillet—don't use pans with plastic parts that melt in the oven.

Ingredients for the Frittata

2 eggs

1/2 cup chopped bell pepper and onions (fresh or frozen and thawed)

2 slices deli ham, thinly sliced and cut into pieces

1 tomato, sliced

1 oz shredded mozzarella cheese

1 tbsp Parmesan cheese, grated

2 tbsp 1% milk

2 tbsp water

Nonstick cooking spray

Salt and pepper

Ingredients for the Toast

1 slice whole-grain toast

1 tbsp cream cheese

continued

Ingredients for the Side Salad

1 cup salad greens   1/2 cup baby carrots
5 cherry tomatoes   1 tsp olive oil
1/2 cucumber, sliced   1 tsp lemon or balsamic vinegar

Directions

1. Heat the oven on broil.
2. Whisk eggs and milk in a bowl and set aside.
3. Heat a small skillet coated with nonstick cooking spray over medium heat and sauté the onions, tomatoes, and peppers until softened, about 5 minutes. Add 1 tablespoon of water as needed to prevent the vegetables from sticking to the pan.
4. Add ham slices, heating until desired crispness; then pour in egg mixture, sprinkle in cheeses and salt and pepper to taste.
5. Cook eggs until done in the center (about 4–5 minutes).
6. While eggs are cooking, combine ingredients for side salad and prepare the toast with cream cheese. Put the pan in the oven (on broil) for about 1 minute (keep an eye on it, as exact broiling time may vary; but the top should be slightly browned when it's done).
7. Use a spatula to loosen the edges of the frittata and then slide it out of the pan onto the serving plate.

Nutrition Facts

Cal 570, Fat 29 g, Fiber 7 g, Sugar 19 g, Protein 37 g, Sodium 610 mg

RD Recommendation: Pasta and Rice

The label for whole-wheat pasta should say 100 percent whole grain and contain at least 3 g of fiber per serving. Skip the white processed rice and opt for whole-grain varieties including brown, wild, red, or brown basmati, as these contain the fiber and nutrients that are often lost in the processing of polished white rice.

Garlic Pasta with Chicken

If you're looking for a quick, satisfying dish, this is it. If you don't care for the taste or texture of pine nuts, you can just leave them out without diminishing the flavor too much.

Ingredients

2 oz dry pasta (we recommend spaghetti noodles)

1/4 tsp minced garlic, dried

1 tsp light butters (we recommend Smart Balance Light)

1/4 tsp Italian seasoning (no salt added)

1/4 cup broccoli

4 oz precooked chicken breast strips

1 tbsp pine nuts

Ingredients for the Salad

1/2 cup baby carrots

1 cup lettuce greens

1 tomato, sliced

1 tbsp balsamic vinaigrette

1 tbsp cranberries

2 tbsp croutons

Directions

1. Boil water and add pasta, cooking according to package instructions. Drain.
2. Add garlic, light butter, Italian seasoning, broccoli, and precooked chicken breast.
3. Keep on low heat for 2–3 minutes.
4. Combine salad ingredients.
5. Place pasta on the plate, top with pine nuts, and serve with side salad.

Nutrition Facts

Cal 570, Fat 16 g, Fiber 7 g, Sugar 15 g, Protein 38 g, Sodium 820 mg

Pizza in a Flash!

This is another great swap for takeout. It's so cheesy and crispy—more like the thin-crust pizzas you get in Italy. Go ahead and experiment. You can replace the ham with pineapple, anchovies, or another favorite topping so long as you keep it low in fat and calories. No arugula on hand? No problem. One of our testers made it with spinach instead and said it was delicious!

Ingredients

1 6½" pita (we recommend whole wheat, though white works)

1 tbsp olive oil

1/2 cup onions and bell peppers, fresh or frozen and thawed

1 plum tomato, sliced (or 8 sliced cherry tomatoes)

1 tbsp Parmesan cheese, grated

1/2 cup arugula, chopped

2 slices deli ham, thinly sliced

2 oz shredded mozzarella cheese

Nonstick cooking spray

Directions

1. Heat oven to 400 degrees F.
2. On a baking sheet coated with nonstick cooking spray, top the pita with olive oil, onions and bell peppers, sliced tomato, and Parmesan and mozzarella cheeses. Place in oven.
3. Heat the ham in a pan coated with nonstick cooking spray over medium heat until crisp.
4. Remove pizza from oven after 8 minutes (when cheese is melted), top with ham, and place in the oven for another 2 minutes.
5. Serve pizza topped with arugula.

Nutrition Facts

Cal 560, Fat 33 g, Fiber 6 g, Sugar 5 g, Protein 25 g, Sodium 850 mg

Pasta Marinara with Grilled Garbanzos

This dish is not only a healthy way to get your carbs and proteins in one shot—it also looks beautiful in the serving dish. It's the perfect dish for a very hungry vegetarian.

Ingredients for the Pasta

1/2 cup fresh basil, chopped

1/2 tsp garlic, minced

2 oz bowtie pasta, dry

1 tbsp toasted pine nuts

1 tbsp Parmesan cheese, grated

1/3 can garbanzo beans

1/2 cup marinara sauce

1 tsp olive oil

Ingredients for the Salad

1 cup mixed salad greens

2 tbsp shredded carrots

1/3 medium cucumber, sliced

1 tsp olive oil

1 tsp lemon juice or to taste

Directions

1. Boil water in pot on stove.
2. Toast garbanzo beans in a small pan with olive oil (about 2–3 minutes or until golden brown).
3. Add pasta to boiling water and cook for about 8–10 minutes.
4. Heat marinara on stove and add chopped basil (or 1 teaspoon ground basil).
5. Drain pasta, mix into marinara sauce, top with garbanzo beans, Parmesan, and toasted pine nuts.
6. Serve pasta dish with tossed salad.

Nutrition Facts

Cal 610, Fat 22 g, Fiber 12 g, Sugar 16 g, Protein 22 g, Sodium 240 mg

Produce: Fresh versus Frozen

Fresh produce is expensive, especially if some spoils before you get a chance to eat it. Frozen fruits and veggies may be a less expensive and more convenient option, especially when your favorites aren't in season.

No concerns about nutrition either. If the produce you're buying isn't locally grown, frozen options often are more nutritious than what's stocked on supermarket shelves. One study by the Centre for Food Innovation at Sheffield Hallam University tested more than thirty-five varieties of produce and found that frozen versions were nutritionally comparable to, if not better than, fresh.[21]

Not all brands are created equal, so be sure to check labels. Some add butter or sauce for flavoring, and frozen fruits often contain added sugar. If it's got a fancy name or a long list of ingredients, it's less likely to be a wise choice.

If You Must . . .

Panda Express Golden Treasure Shrimp

Cal 390, Fat 19 g, Fiber 2 g, Sugar 15 g, Protein 16 g, Sodium 500 mg

Mixed Veggies (side)

Cal 35, Fat 0 g, Fiber 3 g, Sugar 2 g, Protein 2 g, Sodium 260 mg

Panda Express Mushroom Chicken

Cal 220, Fat 13 g, Fiber 1 g, Sugar 4 g, Protein 17 g, Sodium 760 mg

Steamed Rice (side)

Cal 380, Fat 0 g, Fiber 0 g, Sugar 0 g, Protein 7 g, Sodium 0 mg

High sodium levels explain the bloated feeling you get after eating most fast food.

CHAPTER

12 | Discretionary Calories

"Most days it feels like a better idea to grab a Mountain Dew or cappuccino, but that actually makes you feel worse in the long run!"
—Keri, original *Thin in 10* focus group member

To snack or not to snack—that is the million-dollar question. While some studies have shown metabolic benefits of snacking throughout the day, others have found it can lead to weight gain. So the jury is still out on whether you should stick to three meals or have a few snacks in between to (in theory) keep your blood sugar steady. What we can tell you for sure is that everyone's body is different, and the decision to snack should be based on what works best for you. For this reason, the *Thin in 10* Meal Plan allows for up to 200 discretionary calories per day. You may choose to take advantage of these calories every single day or just some days.

In this chapter, we've included some quick and delicious snack options. Many of these are of the grab-and-go variety because we recognize the nature of snacking; when you need a little something, even 10 minutes can seem like a lifetime. The few that require limited preparation are here because we know that sometimes you want something a little more complex in flavor and texture. We've broken up the snacks into two categories: 100 calories, in case you prefer to have two snack breaks per day; and 200 or fewer calories, in case you prefer to have one larger indulgence as, say, a dessert after dinner.

Any calories you drink count toward your snack calorie allowance. As discussed in chapter 6, liquid calories can add up if you're not careful. It's easy to gulp down 150 calories or more in a single serving of a sugary drink or adult beverage. The caution here is that these calories don't leave you feeling very satisfied.

If you are going to imbibe some of your calories, be conscious of serving size since glasses—especially in bars and restaurants—vary widely in volume and may be significantly larger than a recommended 8-ounce serving. Also, when it comes to hard liquor, remember that the higher the "proof," the more calories it has (for example, 100-proof alcohol contains around 125 calories per 1½ ounces, while 80-proof has only 97 calories).

Alrighty. Now that you've got the information you need, here's to happy—and sensible—snacking!

Beverages That Won't Push You Over Your 200-Calorie Limit

Remember, 8 ounces isn't that much; many serving glasses and most cans and bottles hold 16 ounces or more, so if you do decide to sip, stop at 8 ounces to stay under 200 calories. And unless you make it yourself, some of these beverages could contain sugar or added ingredients that could alter the calorie count slightly. The totals below are general estimates:

Drink Calories (per 8 oz)

Vitamin water	50	Margarita	200
Lemonade	140	Rum and Coke	185
Whole milk	150	Wine spritzer	100
Chocolate milk	200	Screwdriver	190
Cola	120	Champagne	156
Orange juice	110	Red wine	192
Sweet tea	120	White wine	150
Caffe latte (whole milk)	180	Gin and tonic	175
Mojito	200		

100-Calorie Snack Ideas

Food	Calories	Fat (g)	Fiber (g)	Sugar (g)	Protein (g)	Sodium (mg)
Fruit and Veggie Snacks						
1 small banana	100	0	3	19	1	0
1 medium apple	100	0	4	23	0	0
1 medium pear	100	0	4	17	1	0
28 grapes	100	0	1	23	1	0
25 baby carrots	100	0	7	12	2	200
3 tbsp raisins	100	0	2	22	1	10
1/4 cup cranberries	100	0	2	.023	0	0
20 cherries	100	0	1	15	1	0
5 dates	100	0	3	22	1	0
3/4 mango	100	0	3	23	1	0
1½ medium nectarine	100	0	3	18	2	0
3 plums	100	0	3	24	2	0
2 medium tangerines	100	0	3	16	1	0
1/2 pomegranate	100	1	6	19	2	0
Sweet and Salty Treats						
1 Simply Well dark chocolate pudding cup	100	1.5	3	13	4	150
1 oz pretzels	100	0	1	1	2	350
11 baked chips	100	4	1	1	0	200
1/2 oz mixed nuts, unsalted	100	7	0	1	3	0
13 almonds, unsalted	100	8	2	1	3	0
1 medium sliced cucumber with 1/4 cup non-fat Greek yogurt, lemon juice, and pepper (to taste)	100	0	3	9	8	20
1 cup broccoli and 3 tbsp hummus	100	4.5	5	0	6	190
3/4 cup edamame	100	4	4	2	9	5
1 cup snow peas and 3 tbsp hummus	100	4.5	4	3	5	170

200-Calorie (or Less) Snack Ideas

2 tbsp salsa and 1 oz baked tortilla chips (such as Tostitos)

Cal 160, Fat 7 g, Fiber 1 g, Sugar 2 g, Protein 2 g, Sodium 350 mg

With very few calories, tomato salsa provides heart-healthy lycopene (an antioxidant that may play a role in preventing various cancers, cardio-vascular disease, and diseases of the eye). Limiting the chips to an ounce is an ideal way to keep your caloric intake within reason and a tasty way to enjoy your zesty, flavorful salsa.

10 olives and 1 thin slice Swiss cheese

Cal 180, Fat 15 g, Fiber 0 g, Sugar 0 g, Protein 6 g, Sodium 650 mg

Sugar-free, this savory snack is a satisfying combination of tangy and salty flavors. Olives offer heart-healthy mono-unsaturated fats—the high oleic acid content has been noted for reducing risk for cardiovascular disease. This snack is perfectly portioned to keep your dietary fats within healthy limits.

1 (1/2 oz) square dark chocolate and 1 medium banana

Cal 180, Fat 5 g, Fiber 4 g, Sugar 25 g, Protein 2 g, Sodium 0 mg

Dark chocolate offers a little decadence, plus some heart-healthy benefits. Along with other important nutrients, the banana offers magnesium and potassium (essential for steady heart rhythm/function), and provides an adequate amount of dietary fiber. Combined, they offer satisfaction in both flavor and satiety to curve your cravings.

2–3 oz turkey and 1 thin provolone cheese slice wrapped in 1 leaf of romaine lettuce

Cal 160, Fat 6 g, Fiber 0 g, Sugar 0 g, Protein 23 g, Sodium 610 mg

Choose low-sodium thinly sliced deli turkey (regular turkey slices can put you at 800–1,000 mg of sodium for this snack alone). Turkey and cheese are a great flavor combination that both satisfies and offers plenty of protein.

6 oz nonfat Greek yogurt, 1 tsp honey, and 1 cup strawberries

Cal 160, Fat 0 g, Fiber 3 g, Sugar 19 g, Protein 16 g, Sodium 65 mg
A low-fat, low-sodium treat, this one is sure to satisfy with a healthy dose of protein and adequate dietary fiber. Since strawberries are so low in calories, you can enjoy a whole cupful of antioxidant-rich berries.

A bowl of Kix cereal

Cal 170, Fat 2 g, Fiber 3g, Sugar 9g, Protein 7g, Sodium 260 mg
Because Kix isn't loaded with sugars, fats, or calories, you can enjoy a tasty bowl-full of cereal. This generous portion provides adequate fiber and protein to keep you satisfied.

2 tbsp Nutella

Cal 200, Fat 11 g, Fiber 1 g, Sugar 21 g, Protein 3 g, Sodium 15 mg
With little protein and fiber to balance its sugar load, this treat is no nutrient superstar. But one delicious spoonful satisfies a sweet tooth and won't put your caloric load over the top.

Peanut butter (2 tsp) & jelly (1 tsp) on a 100-calorie sandwich thin

Cal 190, Fat 6 g, Fiber 6 g, Sugar 6 g, Protein 7 g, Sodium 270 mg
A classic favorite, this PB&J offers enough protein and fiber to satisfy and also provides a heart-healthy source of mono-unsaturated fat. The minimal sugar from the jelly offers sweetness without going overboard.

Plain oatmeal packet (1/2 cup oats) sweetened with honey (1 tsp) and blueberries (1/4 cup)

Cal 190, Fat 3 g, Fiber 5 g, Sugar 10 g, Sodium 0 mg
Oatmeal is a cholesterol-lowering food that really does satisfy. Sweetening your oatmeal with just a bit of honey and fresh berries is the way to go for a delicious, antioxidant-rich snack.

200-Calorie (or Less) Snack Ideas *continued*

Avocado slices on crackers

Cal 190, Fat 12 g, Fiber 6 g, Sugar 0 g, Protein 4 g, Sodium 35 mg

Avocados are a great source of heart-healthy monounsaturated fats. Did you know that 2 tablespoons of avocado is lower in calories than the same amount of butter or cream cheese?

Cucumber slices topped with cream cheese

Cal 140, Fat 10 g, Fiber 3 g, Sugar 7 g, Sodium 95 mg

Cucumbers are the way to go if you're craving cheese. High in water content and low in calories, cucumbers offer a delicate crunch and subtle flavor—a nice balance for the rich tanginess of the cheese.

Egg pizza

Cal 170, Fat 12 g, Fiber 0 g, Sugar 0 g, Protein 14 g, Sodium 290 mg

1 scrambled egg (cooked in a nonstick pan without oil), with 1 tablespoon tomato bruschetta and 1/4 cup shredded mozzarella cheese. One of Jessica's favorite snacks, an egg served up this way is delicious and offers healthy protein, vitamin D, and eye-healthy antioxidants (lutein, zeaxanthin, and lycopene).

Kale crisps with yogurt dip

Cal. 200, Fat 10 g, Fiber 2 g, Sugar 5 g, Protein 14 g, Sodium 85 mg

1½ cups fresh kale, chopped	4 oz nonfat Greek yogurt
2 tsp olive oil	2 tsp lemon juice
1 garlic clove, minced	Pepper

To make, toss and coat the kale with olive oil and garlic, and then toast in oven until crisp. For the yogurt dip, combine nonfat Greek yogurt with lemon juice and add pepper to taste.

Parmesan popcorn

Cal 133, Fat 3 g, Fiber 3.5 g, Sugar 0 g, Protein 5 g, Sodium 152 mg

3 cups of air popped popcorn topped with 4 teaspoons of reduced-fat, grated Parmesan cheese (to add even more flavor, sprinkle 1/2 teaspoon paprika or lemon pepper on top).

If You Must . . .

McDonald's Fruit and Yogurt Parfait

Cal 160, Fat 2 g, Fiber 1 g, Sugar 21 g, Protein 4 g, Sodium 85 mg

If you've just gotta have fast food, this snack isn't going to do you wrong. At under 200 calories, this low-fat parfait is simply low-fat vanilla yogurt, fresh fruit, and a little granola.

Starbucks small coffee and biscotti

Cal 180, Fat 7 g, Fiber 1 g, Sugar 16 g, Protein 4 g, Sodium 125 mg

This snack is not fiber rich and perhaps a little empty caloried. What better way to stay under 200 calories than to enjoy a rich cup of coffee with a biscotti to dip and enjoy slowly at your leisure.

RD Recommendation: Nuts and Fruit

Nuts

Skip the candied varieties and opt for simple roasted, unsalted nuts. Almonds are your best bets for vitamin E, and walnuts are a good source of omega-3s.

Fruit

Eat fresh or frozen fruit whenever possible. We do recommend dates, a dried fruit. Other dried fruits may be okay too, but steer clear if they contain added sugars or fats (dried banana chips are a perfect "unhealthy" dried fruit example).

PART III

Living the *Thin in 10* Life!

13 How to Burn (or Trim) Extra Calories Every Day

Diet and exercise are the pillars of your *Thin in 10* program, but did you know there is a third pillar, something just as essential to your weight-loss efforts as diet and exercise? We call it lifestyle movement. If you've had trouble losing weight in the past despite being virtuous about workouts and food, paying attention to lifestyle movement could be the key to finally losing weight and keeping it off once and for all.

Lifestyle movement refers to activities woven into your day that are too insignificant or short-term to be considered a workout or even a form of exercise. Activities like walking from the kitchen to the living room to hiking up a flight of stairs to standing in line at the grocery store fall into this category. Even little actions like jiggling your foot, twisting a paper clip, and chewing gum count. You probably don't pay much attention to these bits of movement because they are so incidental. Yet they are physical activity, and they do burn calories.

On its own, each smidgen of lifestyle movement burns up a miniscule number of calories. However, tallied up over the course of a day, they account for anywhere from 15 percent to more than 50 percent of daily energy expenditure. Fidgety people who can't sit still burn at the higher end of this range while those who are sluggish burn at the lower range. This means two people of similar size can have a 2,000-calorie burn difference per day depending on how much lifestyle movement they get. Obviously, the mover and shaker is likely to have an easier time dropping pounds than the slower go-er.

Sit and Unfit

Lifestyle movement can be a relatively painless way to ratchet up calorie burn, making it a very effective tool for weight loss, but it's been increasingly engineered out of daily life. Thanks to modern conveniences and labor-saving technology, the average person now spends more than half his or her waking hours sitting. A major shift has also occurred in what most of us do to earn a living. With more than 40 percent of workers employed on farms in the early part of last century, working up a sweat was part of the job. Today, less than 2 percent of the labor force does active farmwork. More than 80 percent of us now sit behind a desk, typically staring at a screen and tapping away at a keyboard for eight or more hours per day.

All this sitting may seem harmless enough because, well, it's so comfy. But in terms of calorie burn, it's a disaster. Sitting at your desk burns about 80 calories an hour. Compare that to standing, which burns about 115 calories an hour. This difference of 35 calorie per hour sounds paltry until you do the math.

"Sitting at your desk burns about 80 calories an hour."

For argument's sake, let's be generous and say you spend about five hours a day rooted to your chair. Over the course of the day, that's a missed opportunity to expend about 175 calories (the equivalent of one 6" pancake, without syrup or butter). Multiply that out for an entire year and it totals nearly 64,000 calories you didn't burn, corresponding to eighteen pounds you either gained or didn't lose. Some studies have found an even greater calorie burn disparity between sitting and standing. In a 2005 Mayo Clinic investigation, the heavier subjects tended to sit more than the leaner ones, who were more

Add Activity 10 Minutes at a Time

Don't believe that adding just a little lifestyle movement can really pay off? Here's an example of how you can benefit from engineering some lifestyle movement into things you do anyway. Add just one activity for an extra calorie hit; or, if they fit into your day without too much effort, add them all. Remember, each of these 10-minute hits can be accumulated over the course of the day—you don't have to do the full 10 minutes all at once.

10 Minutes' Worth of Activity	Calories Burned
Carrying a baby (or grocery bags)	37
Pushing a stroller (or grocery cart)	26
Climbing stairs	85
Sweeping the floor	26
Making beds	21
Washing dishes	24
Watering the lawn/plants	16
Talking on the phone (standing)	19
Helping kids with homework (standing)	21
Walking to the store	49

fidgety and spent an average of two additional hours a day on their feet. The difference translated into 350 calories a day, enough for the heavy people to prevent a gain (or loss) of, or take off, thirty-five pounds a year at least theoretically. How else may sitting contribute to your expanding waistline? Studies show that many people tend to mindlessly snack while sitting and staring into a screen of some sort, eating more and making poor nutritional choices. In short, it's likely that you're not only burning fewer calories when you sit but also taking in more. Not a great combo when your dream is to buy clothes in a smaller size.

Beyond the low caloric expenditure and increased caloric intake, prolonged sitting promotes a lack of whole-body muscle movement. Scientists are becoming increasingly alarmed about what sitting for extended periods of time does to the body, even for dedicated exercisers. It appears that muscle movement and muscle contractions help control important blood fats. After four hours of sitting, the genes and enzymes regulating the amount of glucose and fat in the body start to shut down. Instead, fat in the bloodstream appears to be captured and stored by fat cells throughout the body but especially around organs such as the kidneys. This is a very dangerous place for fat to settle and ups your risk of diabetes, heart disease, and some cancers.

Stand Up for Weight Loss (and Health)

If you've somehow squeezed most of the lifestyle movement out of your daily life, deliberately adding as much movement back as possible can make a huge difference in your weight-loss efforts. Certainly, we're not suggesting you give up on a formal exercise program (please don't!), but racking up at least 10 minutes of additional lifestyle movement per day increases your calorie burn and muscle usage gently over the course of the day. Best of all, the extra effort is barely noticeable.

Add 1 Minute of Activity at a Time

If you want to make it really painless, accumulate ten, 1-minute hits of additional lifestyle activity during the day. These actions are barely noticeable but still effective. Here's an example of ten, 1-minute activities and the associated calorie burn.

1 Minute's Worth of Activity	Calories Burned
Twist a rubber band in your hand	3
Roll a ball with your foot	3
Stand on one leg	1
Tap your pencil	3
Laugh at a couple of jokes	3
Walk to your destination from the far end of the parking lot	6
Do twenty slow squats while talking on the phone	6
Do butt squeezes while stuck in traffic	6
Jog part of the way to a meeting	8
Jiggle your leg	3
Total extra calories burned	*42*

To help you kick-start a lifestyle movement plan, pages 180–185 include fifty-four ways you can easily burn an additional ten calories or more—in some cases a lot more—as you go about your day. None of the strategies is time-consuming. In fact, many actually turn out to be time-savers. Also, nothing here should overtax you physically. Yet over time, they add

"It's like a workout's worth of calories for free."

up to a substantial calorie burn—without you breaking a sweat. It's like a workout's worth of calories for free.

Ten Easy Ways to Trim Calories from Your Diet without Noticing a Thing

The flip side of adding activity into your day is, of course, taking away a few calories here or there. In addition to the tasty, low-calorie recipes in the meal plan chapters, here are some easy ways to cut calories:

Activity	Calories Trimmed
1. Hold the mayo and use mustard on your sandwich instead	90
2. Skip 2 tablespoons of sugar in your morning coffee	32
3. Leave the last five bites on your plate at dinner	250
4. Substitute a baked apple sprinkled with cinnamon and a hint of sugar for a piece of apple pie	290
5. Enjoy a kiddie-size popcorn at the movies instead of a "small" serving	200
6. Make your sandwiches open-faced—leave off the top slice of bread	100
7. Put half a pat of butter on your toast instead of a full pat	50
8. Just say "no thanks" to the samples at the grocery store; tasting that stale piece of cheese isn't worth the extra calories	150
9. Substitute one sugary drink, like soda or juice, with a glass of water (minimum!)	120
10. Use nonstick cooking spray instead of 2 tablespoons of oil	250

54 Ways to Burn Calories

At Home Do This   **Burn This Many Calories**

1. Take 10 minutes to prepare your own meal (see any of our meal chapters for recipes). Besides the bonus calories burned, it gives you control over the number of calories in your meal.   23

2. When you're done eating the delicious meal you prepared yourself, take 10 minutes to clean up the kitchen.   40

3. Do a little permanent press by ironing clothes for 10 minutes. Use your nondominant hand for even more muscle activation.   26

4. Can't find anything to wear? Spend 10 minutes organizing your closet—clean out drawers, donate clothes, stack the shoe rack, and so on.   43

5. Does your yard need a little sprucing up? Spend 10 minutes raking leaves or weeding.   45

6. Do a "clean sweep" of the house and spend 10 minutes putting away toys, clothes, magazines, mail, and so on. Add an extra 20 calories burned if you have to take three or more trips up the stairs.   27

7. Walk the dog for 10 minutes. Don't have a dog? Offer to take the neighbor's dog for a walk or just pretend you have one. In other words, get out and walk around the block!   40

8. Washing windows is a great total-body workout. Do it for 10 minutes to improve the way your windows—and arms—look.   51

9. Hate mopping? Grab a Swiffer Duster and do a quick sweep of the floors for 10 minutes.   28

10. Add several glasses of water a day to your diet. Pour each glass individually so you have to get up every time. Those extra trips, plus the few inevitable extra visits to the bathroom, inch your daily calorie burn up.   20

At Play Do This	Burn This Many Calories
11. Pucker up to turn your partner into a calorie-burning machine! Kiss your man or woman for 7 minutes. Besides burning calories, it can also lead to this . . .	10
12. Massaging your partner for 10 minutes at the end of the day burns bonus calories—and gives you untold bonus points. And that might lead to this….	45
13. Have some fun with your partner doing, well, you know!	34
14. Go clothes shopping. Even if you don't buy anything, searching through racks and trying on clothes for 10 minutes makes it easier to fit into them.	40
15. Turn up the radio and dance like no one is watching during three of your favorite songs.	77
16. Take a 10-minute afternoon catnap to burn extra calories and balance out hunger hormones so you are less likely to have an afternoon snack attack.	15
17. Hide the remote, cut your typical daily TV time in half, and watch your activity level soar.	119
18. Practice good posture all day. In addition to the extra calories used, standing up taller makes you appear 10 pounds thinner.	50
19. Find any excuse to stand on one leg periodically throughout the day, like when you're brushing your teeth or blow-drying your hair. Accumulate a total of 10 minutes.	10
20. Listen to music throughout your day. Studies show that you are more likely to stay in motion—whether tapping your foot to the beat, swaying to the rhythm, or simply moving around a little faster in general.	75
21. Chew gum for 10 minutes.	11

54 Ways to Burn Calories *continued*

With the Kids Do This	Burn This Many Calories
22. Challenge your children to a game of Ultimate Frisbee! A 10-minute game is a good way to get them moving too.	40
23. Put a hula hoop around your hips and start swaying; 10 minutes of this fun pastime is a great way to work your core.	57
24. Play a video game in which you move to keep up with the action on the screen or a game pad.	50
25. Pull out the Monopoly board and allow a few additional calories to pass Go! (Play for 30 minutes.)	51
26. Rather than sitting in the stands as an idle spectator at your kid's sports activities, stand and cheer, walk around to view the game from different angles, and prowl the sidelines for at least an hour of the action.	75
27. Have a tickle session! Studies show that laughing and chasing your little one around for 10 minutes is good for heart health.	20
28. Challenge your tyke to a 10-minute Ping-Pong tournament to bond and burn calories.	68
29. Jump on a trampoline or mini-rebounder for 10 minutes. It's a great way to tone muscles and elevate heart rate.	40
30. Grab some balls or pieces of fruit and start tossing. Juggle for 10 minutes. It's fun even if you never catch a thing.	45
31. Find a piece of sidewalk chalk and a couple of rocks. Play hopscotch for 10 minutes.	57
32. Dust off your old bike and go for a spin around the neighborhood for 10 minutes.	51

Out and About Do This	Burn This Many Calories
33. Use a grocery basket instead of a cart during a 10-minute shopping trip. Bonus: strengthen and tone arm muscles.	40
34. Hike up the escalator instead of simply going along for the ride.	9
35. Accumulate 10 minutes a day of on-the-go grooming, including combing your hair, brushing your teeth, changing outfits, and any other little self-improvement tasks that make you look good.	28
36. Add just 1,000 extra steps per day to your usual activity level; it's a nice stride toward the ultimate goal of taking 10,000 steps per day, which many health experts recommend.	35
37. Add a lap to your usual routine to accumulate 10 extra minutes of movement. Walking from the parking lot into the store? Walk a lap around the lot before going in. Then add a lap around the perimeter of the grocery store or department store before you start shopping.	45
38. Stand rather than sit for 30 minutes while you watch your child's after-school soccer game or gymnastics.	61
39. Take the 10 minutes needed per school day to walk the kids home from the bus stop and carry their backpacks.	40
40. Do a few standing stretches while you wait in line or talk on the phone, for a total of 5 minutes throughout the day.	22
41. Near a park bench? Do a short circuit of dips, push-ups, and step-ups for a total of 5 minutes.	45
42. Walk around with shopping bags or a full purse. Doing this even for 10 minutes a day makes a difference.	28

54 Ways to Burn Calories *continued*

At Work Do This	Burn This Many Calories
43. For at least 5 minutes, jog from one appointment or errand to the next. You'll get there faster and burn calories at a 37 percent higher rate compared with walking.	40
44. Swap out your desk chair for a stability ball to sit up straighter and have a little more fun at work. Do this for four hours and the additional calorie burn becomes significant.	80
45. Better yet, stand up 10 minutes of every hour for half your workday (four hours). It's a great way to tone muscles and improve your blood profile.	116
46. Fidget at your desk intermittently throughout your eight-hour workday. Tap your foot or pencil, play with a rubber band, or jiggle your leg—anything to keep moving.	200
47. Walk to your coworker's desk on the other side of the building instead of sending an e-mail. You'll probably get back the 5 minutes per day this takes by getting your answers a lot quicker!	16
48. Use a speakerphone or headset and take phone calls only while pacing. It's a great way to focus your concentration and burn an extra 68 calories during a 10-minute phone call.	68

At Work Do This	Burn This Many Calories

49. To burn calories and tone up your legs, skip the elevator every time your trip is three flights or less.   12

50. To jack up your stair-climbing calorie count by 55 percent, take them two at a time. Double stepping those same three flights burns about 19 calories—and seriously sculpts your glutes!   19

51. A study commissioned by the American Council on Exercise found that workers dressed in business casual clothing instead of more formal wear burned more calories in a day because they were more likely to get up and move around. So if you've got the option, ditch your Spanx and heels for a casual-dress outfit.   25

52. Roll a tennis ball or a racquet ball around with your bare foot as you work. Do this for 10 minutes with your foot discreetly under your desk so no one notices (and it feels great under the arches of your feet after a day in heels).   26

53. Making copies? Don't send someone else to do it for you—burn the calories yourself!   20

54. Volunteer to pick up lunch for the office. That 10-minute walk to and from the deli and the workout from carrying the food back helps burn off part of your lunch.   55

14 | Skinny Sleep

Throughout this book, we've touted the idea of changing your life 10 little minutes at a time. We truly believe that the 10 minutes it takes to exercise, prepare a meal, take a deep breath, or engineer a little extra movement into your day can absolutely transform your body—and your life. Sleep is the one activity where we ask you to ignore this Rule of 10. Read on and we'll explain.

Mirror-Image Trends

Until the mid-1900s, the average person slept around nine hours a night. Then, about thirty years ago, experts noticed that the average number of hours slumbered nightly was trending downward. In the 1990s, experts noted that the typical night's sleep had slipped to just under eight hours. By the time the National Sleep Foundation performed a comprehensive nationwide survey in 2008, the majority of adults in the United States reported sleeping just 6 hours and 40 minutes per night.[22]

Experts also noticed that as the number of sleep hours shrunk, waistlines expanded. The number of obese people in the United States has risen a belt-busting 214 percent since the middle of the last century. In 1950, about 10 percent of the population was considered obese. In 2012 about 34 percent of the population is considered obese. This figure does not include the additional 30 percent of the population considered merely overweight. Study after study began to associate lack of sleep and larger size, including one investigation done by Columbia University in New York that reviewed the sleeping habits and body weight of more than 18,000 people. In this study, those who got by on less than four hours of sleep a night were a whopping 73 percent more likely to be obese than people who slumbered seven to nine hours nightly—and even those who caught six hours were 23 percent more likely to be obese. On the other hand, people who averaged ten hours in the land of nod were 11 percent less likely to be obese.[23]

Some scientists now suspect that the opposing trends of less sleep and more body fat are no mere coincidence. There appears to be a strong biological basis for the link. The Columbia researchers, for instance, say sleep deprivation disrupts levels of gherlin and leptin, two of the major hormones that regulate hunger and appetite. When you skimp on sleep, your body reacts much the same way as if you've skipped a meal: Your leptin levels fall as your gherlin levels shoot up. This triggers hunger, which in turn triggers overeating, and that of course leads to weight gain.

"When you skimp on sleep, your body reacts much the same way as if you've skipped a meal."

Studies done at Bristol University in the United Kingdom confirm that people who sleep less than five hours a night have 15 percent less leptin in their bloodstream and 15 percent more ghrelin. They found that these hormonal changes do even more damage by signaling the body to put the brakes on metabolism and cling to fat stores more tenaciously.[24]

Research indicates that some people are more susceptible to weight gain with hormone fluctuations than others and that for some people, even one bad night can be a nightmare for their diet. If you've ever spent a sleepless night followed by a day where you couldn't seem to satisfy your hunger, then you've experienced this effect.

Other recent studies indicate that sleeplessness throws off the body's biological clocks, or circadian rhythms. When the circadian rhythms for glucose and insulin regulation are disturbed, it can lead to faulty metabolism, insulin resistance, and weight gain.[25] Still other studies have found that a sleep deficit can spike up levels of cortisol, a hormone that among other tasks regulates how the body uses energy. Sleeping less than four hours a night may lead to elevated cortisol levels that peak late in the day; high evening cortisol levels have been linked to insulin resistance and a higher body mass index.[26]

Not all experts are convinced that good sleep is helpful in reaching a healthier weight, but from an evolutionary standpoint, the connection makes sense. Our early cave-dwelling ancestors would have benefited from a metabolic regulatory system that drove them to sleep less, eat more, and hold on to greater amounts of fat during the summer months when the days were longer and food was plentiful in order to prepare for the cold, dark winter months when food was scarce. However, now that we've evolved into a species of chronically sleep-deprived desk dwellers with ready access to an ever-abundant food supply, this biological mechanism works against us by contributing to weight problems.

"Quality of sleep is also important."

All this evidence leads us to believe good sleep is an essential part of your *Thin in 10* weight-loss plan. If these twin epidemics do indeed go hand in hand, then part of a good weight-loss strategy would be to spend more time in dreamland to support everything else you're doing to reach your goals.

How Much Sleep Is Enough?

We don't mean to suggest that sleep is a substitute for eating right and moving your body more. Far from it. Our point is that good sleep is just one more weapon to help you win the battle of the bulge. If you're serious about weight loss and total body transformation, the holistic approach, which includes getting adequate shut-eye, is the way to go. It's worth a try especially if you are a chronic under-sleeper. You may find that more slumber helps control the urge to binge and increases your will to eat healthy food and exercise on a regular basis.

So how much should you be sleeping? Well, we can't give you a magic number. No one can tell you for certain how many hours of sleep you should get per night in order to keep extra pounds at bay or for health in general. For many reasons, the amount of sleep required for weight maintenance and better health appears to be different for different groups of people and for each individual specifically. To complicate matters, quality of sleep is also important. You may lie in bed for a full eight hours but toss and turn for four of them. Despite your best effort, you wake up feeling exhausted, and with your hormones thrown out of balance.

Based on current research, the answer seems to be that getting less than seven hours of sleep on a regular basis is likely to send you down a path toward weight gain. Beyond the hormonal changes, observational studies report that people who wake up tired and have to drag themselves through their day tend to make bad food choices. Often, when they're better rested, they're less likely to reach for sweets and high-carbohydrate, high-calorie snacks to provide energy.

Incidentally, it appears regularly sleeping more than nine or ten hours a night may cause hormone imbalances and weight gain. (Studies also vary on what the exact maximum sleep number is.) So the sweet spot for sweet dreams is probably somewhere between seven and nine hours for most people.

If you find that you're already sleeping plenty, or you increase your sleep but after a few weeks still feel sloggy and groggy when you wake up, it's worth checking in with a doctor. You may have an undiagnosed sleep problem that needs to be addressed. Read on for some tips and strategies for better sleep.

Snooze to Lose

Our better-sleep tips are based on recommendations from the National Sleep Foundation (a great resource for anything to do with sleep or lack of thereof):

Keep a regular sleep schedule. Since sleep is regulated by circadian rhythms, it's important to maintain a consistent bedtime and wake-time schedule, even on the weekends. Doing so reinforces your circadian functions so you're more likely to be primed for sleep at the right time and

Give Your Bedroom a Makeover for Better Rest

Not only is preparing your body important for great sleep but so is prepping your bedroom—where all the slumber magic happens. Here are five easy ways to make over your bedroom to improve your chances of a good night's rest:

1. *Clear out the clutter.* This is probably the easiest way to open up space and help channel some relaxing energy into your bedroom—and it won't cost a thing! (In fact, you may find some money during your cleaning process.) Toss or donate anything you haven't used in at least a month, and be sure to put items that don't belong in your bedroom in their proper place. (Kids' toys, Fido's flea collar, and unused exercise equipment are so not sexy.)

2. *Take out the TV.* Okay, we know you like to fall asleep to the late show, and we aren't saying you can't watch TV at night, but removing your TV from the bedroom reduces your exposure to light, and it just may help spice up your love life. Studies show couples who don't have a TV in the boudoir have more sex.

3. *Don a sleep mask.* Believe it or not, even the slight light from your alarm clock or computer charger could be affecting your sleep. Wearing a sleep mask can help you block out all light sources and improve your chances of getting deep rest. (We love lavender-scented masks to enhance the relaxation response.) Can't stand your eyes being covered while you sleep? Be sure to turn all clocks around, cover your chargers, and use blackout shades to block out all sources of light.

4. *Consider changing colors.* You don't have to redecorate everything, but painting your bedroom a cool color (like light blue or gray) could have calming effects on your body at night. Think of your bedroom as a sanctuary and try to decorate it as such.

5. *Open the windows for at least 10 minutes a day.* Consider adding a few plants (ferns or spider or bamboo plants are best) to improve the clean air in your bedroom to help lessen your body's possible reaction to indoor allergens commonly found in the bedroom.

wake up without hitting the snooze half a dozen times. And no, you can't "catch up on" or bank sleep by snoozing later on the weekends to make up for late nights and early mornings during the week.

Learn to relax. A warm bath, classical music, or a soothing cup of caffeine-free tea right before you hit the sack can help you drift off to sleep more easily. Keep your bath warm rather than scalding hot. There's some evidence to suggest that hot temperatures send the body signals to stay awake. Even spending just 5–10 minutes practicing a breathing technique, such as inhaling for ten counts, and exhaling for ten counts, can help your mind switch off and prepare your body for sleep. And stressful activities like paying bills, catching up on e-mails, or texting should be avoided for at least an hour before bedtime to give your mind a chance to wind down.

Lights out. Avoid bright lights for at least an hour before bedtime too, as light has been shown to disrupt sleep circadian rhythms. In particular, avoid modern-day "blue light" emanating from electronics such as computers, iPads, and cell phones. These have been shown to be especially sleep disruptive. Instead, create a sleep-conducive environment that is dark, quiet, comfortable, and cool.

Noises off. Turn off the blaring TV and shut the windows so you aren't bothered by outside sounds. If your partner snores, request that he or she make a doctor's appointment to address it. Consider earplugs or a white-noise machine to block out all distracting noises that might keep you up or wake you up too early.

Make your bed comfy. If you haven't replaced your mattress, pillow, or sheets in years, consider whether it's time for a change. Find a sleep set that matches your personal preference—some beds even allow you to choose one level of firmness on your side while your partner chooses another. Don't let a caved-in mattress or a lumpy pillow be the reason you don't sleep well.

Don't use your bedroom for an office. Your bedroom is for sleep and sex only. Banishing your computer and filing cabinet to another area of your home sends the message that your bedroom is a sanctuary for sleep.

Limit eating. Going to sleep on a full stomach can be uncomfortable, especially if you eat foods that cause heartburn. Avoid caffeine for at least six hours before bedtime and, in general, avoid fluids that might prompt nighttime trips to the bathroom. However, if that isn't an issue, you may find it soothing to sip a cup of warm milk or caffeine-free tea before lights-out.

Exercise early. People who exercise tend to get better sleep. However, doing our Simple Strength routine (see chapter 4) right before bedtime is not likely to induce sleep. On the other hand, studies show that stretching may help you get to sleep faster, so try the 10-Minute Stretch routine (see chapter 7) if you have trouble sleeping.

No smoking. We don't have to explain the thousands of reasons why you shouldn't be smoking. However, if you haven't quit yet, make sure you don't smoke during the last few hours before bedtime. Nicotine, like caffeine, is a stimulant. Taken close to bedtime, it can keep you awake or disrupt sleep. And certainly never smoke in bed when you feel drowsy!

Avoid alcohol. Many people believe a few glasses of wine are just the thing to help them get to sleep, but alcohol actually induces poor sleep, nightmares, and nighttime waking. If you must have a glass of wine, drink it with dinner so it clears your system before you're ready to go to sleep.

Check in with your doctor. If you experience chronic sleep problems, pills are not the answer. Instead talk to your doctor about what might be going on. Consider keeping a sleep diary to show your doctor. If there's an underlying problem, your doctor may send you to a sleep specialist.

Wrap-Up

As we've just discussed, sleep may just be the missing link in your weight-loss efforts. At the very least, getting a good night's rest makes it easier to face the challenges of the coming day. It's easier to make good eating choices and embrace exercise when you aren't exhausted. This is one aspect of the program that helped both of us tremendously. Our focus group members also commented on how adequate sleep was one of the most surprising—and effective—strategies of the *Thin in 10* program.

CHAPTER

15

It's Not Just Physical: The Mental Side of Weight Loss

Think about the times you've successfully stuck to a sensible diet, your exercise routine worked like clockwork, and you even lost a few pounds. There probably wasn't anything particularly magical about the diet or workout program you followed compared to the times you failed. Every time you made it work there was one common denominator: Your head was in the game.

We acknowledge the huge mental component of weight loss and have done our best to structure our program to remove the main obstacles, including, and especially, time—10 minutes is all we ask! However, we know that sometimes even when all the stars are aligned, you just don't feel like getting off your duff or putting down that ice-cream scoop. For times like these, you need a special plan of attack so you don't veer too far off course.

Over the years, we've spoken with clients and readers (including those in our *Thin in 10* focus group) to determine which situations were most likely to have them reaching for a box of cookies or hitting the snooze button instead of lacing up their sneakers. Certain pitfalls seem to be universal. In addition to sharing the following six common scenarios where wherewithal tends to be low, we offer some strategies for pushing through the tough times.

Scenario 1: Keeping the Drive Alive

While everyone knows that exercise is good for you, it seems no one understands why it's so hard for most of us to get motivated to do it. That's a question for the ages.

A common pattern we see is a person who starts out gung ho. At first, we have to hold her back from hitting it hard for an hour every day. Magically, she finds that big gap in her schedule and enthusiastically uses it to burn calories and sculpt muscles. Then, in a few months, weeks, or even days, she can't seem to find the time to squeeze in a workout. Just as magically as it opened, that schedule gap seems to disappear into the ether.

Of course, it's not really time expanding and contracting here. It's motivation. It starts out strong, then fizzles. Because we know that everyone inevitably goes through periods where they're less inspired to perspire, the trick is to keep the motivation fires burning for as long as possible.

> "People who keep a journal lose up to twice as much weight as those who don't."

Keeping a workout journal can help fan the flames of inspiration. Indeed, we believe journaling your daily workouts (and diet) is a key component to any successful weight-loss journey. This powerful tool helps you maximize your weight loss and stay inspired along the way. According to the researchers at Kaiser Permanente's Center for Health Research, people who keep a journal lose up to twice as much weight as those who don't.[29]

When you record your workouts and meals in a journal, you can look back at the end of each day, week, and month and see your accomplishments on paper or a screen. This can inspire you to work even harder. Because you can see proof of what you've actually done versus what you remember or imagined, it keeps you honest. You may think that you're working out four times a week only to flip through your log and discover that you've been overestimating your efforts. Besides, who wants to stare at blank spaces?

There are dozens of free online fitness journals and plenty of paper ones too. If you choose to create your own log, either on paper or a computer, consider including the following information.

Once a week, write down the following:
• your body weight
• any measurements you track
• your goals for the week
• your long-term goals

> "Just about any food can fit into your diet in moderation."

Each day, write down the following:
• details of your workout, including which exercises you did, level of intensity, how you felt, and notes for future changes
• a record of what you ate and drank, including time of day, estimated portions, how you felt, and changes you'd like to make

Scenario 2: The Unhinged Binge

Sooner or later, everyone feels the urge to splurge on their favorite foods. Your urge might build up over a couple of days or hit suddenly as you pass by a bakery that sells éclairs. Some women say it's harder to resist overeating at certain points in their menstrual cycles, while others cite stress, anxiety, and boredom as reliable binge triggers.

An occasional date with a pint of ice cream probably won't set you back in any permanent sense, but if you find yourself undermining your success again and again with too many trips to the fridge or the drive-through, you need to tackle your issues.

First, make sure you haven't gone overboard on deprivation. Our eating plan is sensible and flexible and includes 200 discretionary calories per day. You shouldn't feel like you're starving yourself, nor should you banish all your favorite foods from the menu. Remember, just about any food can fit into your diet in moderation. If you really crave an item that's not included in the plan, consider adding it back in, in reasonable portions.

Thin in 10 is a plan for life so feel free to make sensible, reasonable adjustments to make it work for you. Even if you go slightly over the allotted calorie count for a few days, that's not a deal breaker. Often that'll be enough to satisfy you and prevent you from going off an eating cliff. It's far better than sliding into an all-out binge.

For urges that are for no food in particular and every food in general, try a more mindful way of eating. The term *mindfulness* means staying in the moment with absolute focus on the here and now, without passing judgment. Mindlessness is just the opposite; it means you aren't paying attention to what you're doing and probably have some negative self-talk looping through your brain. Learning to become more mindful overall can translate to a more mindful way of eating. Likewise, learning to relax can help you become more mindful.

When researchers at the Fred Hutchinson Cancer Research Center in Pennsylvania quizzed 303 people about their activity and eating habits, then cross-referenced them to see which groups had the most insight into why they ate and what they ate, it turned out that the yoga devotees were more aware of the social and emotional reasons they reached for a honey-glazed than the average couch potato. Interestingly, they were even more in tune with food than the folks who walked into the same gym but headed for the treadmill, bike, or weight room instead of the yoga studio.[27]

Presumably, couch potatoes, runners, and cyclists are just as concerned as the yogis with how their clothes fit, but they seem to focus on more pragmatic weight-loss strategies such as counting calories and portion sizes versus the feelings that may trigger eating. These are separate skills. When you practice mindful eating, you eat because you're actually hungry versus eating because you're being emotional, distressed, or bored, or because a candy dish is within reach. You also increase body awareness, specifically a sensitivity to hunger.

So if you find yourself caught in a regular cycle of mindless munching, review the previous three days of your health journal to look for patterns and triggers. This alerts you to circumstances where mindfulness can help you get through without blowing your diet. You might try a simple mindfulness tactic such as eating more slowly and truly savoring each bite. Turn off the TV, the computer, the iPad, and the phone; take your plate to the dining room table and pay full attention to what's at the end of your fork or spoon. These simple strategies can help you become more mindful about what you eat and teach you to enjoy smaller portions of your favorite foods.

We also suggest doing the stretch routine found in chapter 7 at a time of day when your thoughts frequently turn to food and indulgence. Like yoga, the act of stretching can have a deeper effect than simply making you more flexible. It's also been shown to help you feel more relaxed and in tune with your body—more mindful. This is why stretching during a weak moment can help you stay focused and in control.

> "Stretching during a weak moment can help you stay focused and in control."

While you should still watch your portions and eat well, adding mindfulness to your willpower toolkit helps you build positive relationships with food and eating. It gives you that little extra edge you sometimes need when you're wrestling with self-control.

Scenario 3: Too Stressed for Success

Most of us don't reach for a carrot after a fight with our partner or a rough day at work. High amounts of stress usually bring on the cravings for anything with lots of calories, fat, carbs, and salt. Eating junk food seems to soothe the soul and calm the mind. For some reason, stress is also a common reason people abandon their workouts—even though burning off a little adrenaline is the thing most likely to make them feel better.

Stress eaters can definitely benefit from the mindfulness strategies we've already discussed, but when you're vibrating with emotions and all you want to do is take to your bed with a box of cookies, it's difficult to stay focused and in the moment. This is when it pays to stop, take a deep breath, and reboot.

We mean literally stop and take a deep breath when stress gets in the way of doing the right thing for your health. Long, slow, deep breaths that originate from the belly encourage full oxygen exchange; that is, the beneficial trade of incoming oxygen for outgoing carbon dioxide. Not surprisingly, this type of breathing slows the heartbeat and can lower or stabilize blood pressure—exactly the effects of stress you want to reverse. Once you're past the initial stress response, you can think more clearly. It's easier to see why eating that entire box of cookies might not be the best idea in the long run and that going for a walk is.

For times of overwhelming stress, we recommend learning a simple technique known as belly breathing. It's easy to learn and has an instant relaxation effect.

Belly Breathing

- If possible, find a quiet place—at least when you are first learning this technique. Sit, lie, or stand in a comfortable position.
- Place one hand on your belly just below your ribs and the other hand on the center of your chest.
- Breathe deeply through your nose as you let your belly push your lower hand out. Your chest should remain still.
- Purse your lips and exhale, using the hand on your belly to gently assist you in pushing all the air out.
- Take three to ten slow, deep belly breaths. Feel the stress melt away.

Scenario 4: The Lonesome Loser

One of the most unexpected obstacles many of us encounter at the beginning of our weight-loss mission is other people. You might find that your loved ones don't support your efforts. Worse, they may try to sabotage them. Or you might find it disheartening to be surrounded by people who don't see your goals as important; they don't try to trip you up, but they're not exactly cheerleaders either. For some of us, it's definitely harder to go it alone.

Although weight loss is a personal journey and no one can do the work for you, we believe that having a strong support system is one of the golden rules of weight loss. Because we tend to be our own worst critics, it helps to have someone on the sidelines offering encouragement, perspective, and positive reinforcement. If you happen to have a bad day or a little slip, it's nice to have someone there to pick you up and dust you off. That person may also be better at understanding the reasons for your setbacks than you.

The best way to get support? Ask for it. Start by having a meeting with your family and friends to let them know what your goals are and the kind of support you would like. You could, for example, ask that certain areas of your house or the workplace be designated as no-junk-food zones. You could ask for help preparing meals, clearing the decks for your 10 minutes of exercise, or switching a particularly fattening daily ritual to one that doesn't involve food. Whatever you think would help make your efforts more successful, ask for help in making it happen.

A really effective strategy is to enlist those close to you to join you in on the *Thin in 10* program. You've heard that misery loves company. We prefer to say that success loves company. When you put it that way, it's a much easier sell. If you've got partners, you're more likely to work up a sweat and less likely to overindulge. Our one caveat here is that if they fall off the wagon, make sure you still hold on tight. Yes, it's nice to have others with whom you can share the experience, but if they can't stick with the program, be prepared to keep going on your own.

> "It's nice to have someone there to pick you up and dust you off."

Joining a support group or organization may also be helpful. Nearly every community has a walking group or a weight-loss support group you can join. There are certainly plenty listed online. We invite you to join the conversation at www.thinin10.com. Some people do well with an online group because it's anonymous; they find it a lot easier to admit their real weight, their ultimate goals, and their shortcomings to strangers they're not likely to bump into at the grocery store. Plus, at this point in the book, we're not strangers anymore, right? Let us help you through your journey—log on and share your story, struggles, and successes so we can cheer you on!

Scenario 5: Hitting the Wall

Few things in life are more frustrating than when you have been cruising along doing everything right, losing weight steadily, and then bam—your metabolism slams on the brakes and your weight doesn't budge for weeks at a time. It's tempting to give up and walk away—straight toward the fridge. But nearly everyone who takes on the challenge of changing their body and their life encounters the dreaded dieter's plateau.

It's hard to predict when it will hit or how long it will last, but experts theorize that weight plateaus are caused by your body reaching a weight "set point" and then refusing to budge unless you really force the issue. It surprises us that there's so little research on the topic. We can only offer suggestions based on what we've tried ourselves and that others have told us helped jump-start their weight loss once again.

Calorie confusion is one method you can use to jolt the body back into weight-loss mode. It's based on the theory that your body is smart but easily confused. For example, it knows you've been following the 1,500 calorie *Thin in 10* meal plan for a while so it decides to settle in at a certain set point of weight loss. But you can throw it a curveball by altering your calorie intake from one day to the next.

> "Your body is smart but easily confused."

Upping calorie intake by 200 calories for two days then dipping 200 calories below the 1,500-calorie threshold for two days and continuing this up and down cycle for several weeks keeps your body guessing and should give it a jolt back into the fat-melting business.

You can also practice calorie confusion with exercise either separately or at the same time you practice dieting calorie confusion. Something as simple as working out at a different time of day, splitting up your 10-minute sessions if you normally do them together, or doing them back to back if you normally spread them out may be enough to startle your body back into the calorie-burning business. A simple change like switching up many of the variations of the exercises may also get the scales tipping in your favor once again.

If you try tweaking your exercise and diet program and you're still in a holding pattern, flip back to chapter 13 and read up on how burning lifestyle calories can make a difference. Many people who are dedicated exercisers and who watch what they eat sit at a desk all day without so much as shifting in their chairs. Even if you just commit to standing for several hours a day, the calorie burn could add up. Sitting at your desk burns about 80 calories an hour, whereas standing burns about 115. Over the course of the day, that's an opportunity to use up an extra 175 calories. Without any extra time and minimal effort, this may be enough to get the pounds to start melting off again.

That's just one example of how adding more movement to your lifestyle could potentially help you drop a clothing size. You can skim through the chapters and find numerous ways to tweak your calorie burn. A little here and a little there has the potential to make a big difference in your efforts. For that matter, flip to chapter 14, Skinny Sleep, and review our recommendations on sleep. A little extra shut-eye to help balance out hunger and fat-storage hormones might be what's lacking in your weight-loss efforts.

Finally, take a good hard look at yourself. Have you really been as virtuous as you say you've been? Let's go to the videotape, or at least that food and workout journal we've mentioned. If you haven't been losing weight or if you've even been gaining weight, start keeping a journal and pore through it to root out what's truly going on. This does two things for you: It makes you think twice before reaching for that second cookie, and it helps you see what typical eating and movement patterns emerge.

Scenario 6: Instant-Gratification Junkie

You do your first workout and then run to the mirror to see if you look thinner. Sound familiar? It's human nature to hope changes happen quickly. But nature doesn't always cooperate. While wanting instant gratification is understandable in our fast-paced society, not receiving it is often an excuse to give up.

To manage expectations, set up those stepping-stone goals we talked about earlier in this chapter. This allows you to focus on the here and now, rather than a future that can't come soon enough. Instead of obsessing about your end game, setting lots of small, easily reached milestones can renew your sense of accomplishment over and over again. That doesn't mean you give up or forget about your ultimate goals; it just means you inch closer and closer to them without experiencing so much frustration.

> "Setting lots of small, easily reached milestones can renew your sense of accomplishment."

Frankly, sometimes you do need to adjust your expectations. We know that a lot of diet and weight-loss products promise overnight success without any effort on your part. Trust us, that's just marketing. As far as we know, there is no pill, potion, or product that can transform your body overnight or even in one week. That includes plastic surgery.

One hard truth about weight loss: It takes time. You'll feel differences right away and maybe even see changes after the very first workout (for example, stretching may allow you to stand up taller, which makes you look taller instantly). But expect it to take four to eight weeks before you see any real differences in your body, assuming you stick consistently with both the diet and exercise portions of this program. Sometimes in the beginning it is possible to lose five pounds overnight—but that's just water weight. Your body certainly won't lose at that pace for very long. Making real, lasting changes takes patience, dedication, and a healthy dose of reality.

It may also help to keep track of your progress in a number of different ways. Besides checking your weight on the scale, which is often the last number to budge, you can take measurements. Notice the difference in how your clothes fit, plot changes in resting heart rate and blood pressure, or even collect compliments. The more things you track, the more likely you are to find tangible evidence that you really are making progress.

Above all, resist the shortcuts. Our program is built on the idea that numerous smaller changes that you can live with for the rest of your life are always more effective than drastic changes you can deal with for only short periods of time.

Wrap-Up

Do you see yourself in any of the scenarios in this chapter? Many of our focus group members sure did. By using our tips and strategies, they were able to avoid most of the pitfalls they encountered on their road to successful weight loss. If you ever feel discouraged, remember this: Everyone faces challenges, setbacks, and roadblocks when trying to lose weight and improve health. Nothing is insurmountable. Stay focused on your goals. Picture how great you will look and feel when you achieve them. We know you can do it.

Final Thoughts

The Japanese word *kaizen* describes small, incremental changes that over time add up to big improvements. In other words, little changes really can change everything. This philosophy is embodied in our *Thin in 10* plan.

We can't stress enough that this is just the start of your journey. We hope you take all the tips, advice, and information that we've shared with you here and apply it to your life, your way.

The information in these chapters is a lot to digest, so take it in one bite at a time. Start simple. Start small. But do get started. A body in motion tends to stay in motion. And if you fall off the wagon, pick yourself right back up and get going again.

> "It's a plan you can use for the rest of your life."

Throughout this book, we've asked you to make small, incremental changes to your lifestyle that lead to a happier, healthier life—and of course a fitter, firmer, and thinner body. Most important, because the plan is easy to follow, it's a plan you can use for the rest of your life. Follow our routines and you can finally get off the merry-go-round of losing and gaining weight and keep the body you've always wanted. No more New Year's resolutions to drop ten pounds. No more frantic diets a month before swimsuit season. No more wishing you could fit into the next size down. You will always be where you want to be but without the starvation, deprivation, and sacrifice you've experienced with other weight-loss programs.

But as you probably realize by now, this is no quick fix. Nothing happens without your dedication and hard work. Results don't come overnight either. Here again, it's the *kaizen* philosophy: The sum of many small improvements equals one large improvement.

We're confident that once you embrace the workouts, meal plan, and lifestyle changes we've laid out for you, you really can transform your body and then maintain the transformation. Along the way we hope you build supreme confidence and feel more in control of other aspects of your life as well. And if you're ever ready to move beyond our plan to explore longer workouts, different recipes, or further lifestyle changes, we applaud you and say, "Go for it!" Our hope is that we've started you down the right path. Your job is to keep heading in that direction.

Before we leave you, we'd like to say congratulations for choosing to do something great for yourself. You deserve it. Also, we'd like to extend an invitation to join us on www.thinin10.com and tell us where you are starting, where you'd like to go, and how we can continue to help you get there. We're here for you. So is the rest of the *Thin in 10* community. Thank you for reading. We can't wait to continue our relationship with you online.

Notes

Chapter 1: Your 10-Minute Exercise Plan

1. Erin E. Kershaw and Jeffrey S. Flier, "Adipose Tissue as an Endocrine Organ," *JCEM* 89 (2004): 2548–56.
2. Jonathan P. Little, Adeel S. Safdar, Geoffrey P. Wilkin, Mark A. Tarnopolsky, and Martin J. Gibala, "A Practical Model of Low-Volume High-Intensity Interval Training Induces Mitochondrial Biogenesis in Human Skeletal Muscle: Potential Mechanisms," *Journal of Physiology*, 2010.
3. Lewis et al, "Metabolic Signatures of Exercise in Human Plasma," *Science Translational Medicine* 2, no. 33 (May 26, 2010): 33,
4. U. Wisløff, T. I. Nilsen, W. B. Drøyvold, S Mørkved, S. A. Slørdahl, and L. J. Vatten, "A Single Weekly Bout of Exercise May Reduce Cardiovascular Mortality: How Little Pain for Cardiac Gain? 'The HUNT study, Norway,'" *European Journal of Preventive Cardiology* 13, no. 5 (Oct. 2006): 798–804.

Chapter 2: The 10-Minute Walk

5. Melinda L. Irwin, Yutaka Yasui, Cornelia M. Ulrich, Deborah Bowen, Rebecca E. Rudolph, Robert S. Schwartz, Michi Yukawa, Erin Aiello, John D. Potter, Anne McTiernan, "Effect of Exercise on Total and Intra-abdominal Body Fat in Postmenopausal Women: A Randomized Controlled Trial," *Journal of the American Medical Association* 2003; 289, no. 3 (2003): 323–30.
6. James O. Hill, Holly R. Wyatt, George W. Reed, and John C. Peters, "Obesity and the Environment: Where Do We Go from Here?" *Science* 299, no. 5608 (February 7, 2003): 853–55.
7. Yasuyo Hijikata and Seika Yamada, "Walking Just after a Meal Seems to Be More Effective for Weight Loss Than Waiting for One Hour to Walk after a Meal," *International Journal of General Medicine* 4 (2011): 447–50.

Chapter 3: Cardio QUICK

8. Angelo Tremblay, Jean-Aimé Simoneau, Claude Bouchard, "Impact of Exercise Intensity on Body Fatness and Skeletal Muscle Metabolism," *Metabolism* 43, no. 7 (July 1994): 814–18.
9. Izumi Tabata, Kouji Nishimura, Motoki Kouzaki, Yuusuke Hirai, Futoshi Ogita, Motohiko Miyachi, and Kaoru Yamamoto, "Effects of Moderate-Intensity Endurance and High-Intensity Intermittent Training on Anaerobic Capacity and VO2max," *Medicine & Science in Sports & Exercise* 28, no. 10 (October 1996): 1327–30.

Chapter 4: Simple Strength

10. L. S. Nagamatsu, T. C. Handy, C. L. Hsu, M. Voss, T. Liu-Ambrose. "Resistance Training Promotes Cognitive and Functional Brain Plasticity in Seniors with Probable Mild Cognitive Impairment," *Archives of Internal Medicine* 172, no. 8 (2012): 666.

Chapter 5: The 10-Minute Total Body Circuit

11. John Porcari, Kirsten Hendrickson, and Carl Foster, with Mark Anders, "Drop and Give Me 20!" *ACE Fitness Matters* 14, no. 4 (2008): 7–9.

12. Thomas S. Lyons, James W. Navalta, , Mark A. Schafer, Scott W. Arnett, James C. Sivley, Kyle S. Livesay, "Comparative Analysis of Heart Rate during Circuit Training Compared with Different Cardiovascular Training Apparatus," *Medicine & Science in Sports & Exercise* 43, no. 5 (May 2011): 404.

13. T. S. Church, C. K. Martin, A. M. Thompson, C. P. Earnest C. R. Mikus and S. Blair, "Changes in Weight, Waist Circumference and Compensatory Responses with Different Doses of Exercise among Sedentary, Overweight Postmenopausal Women," *PLoS ONE* 4, no. 2 (2009): e4515. doi:10.1371/journal.pone.0004515.

Chapter 6: Core & More

14. P. R. Francis, F. W. Kolhorst, M. Pennuci, R. S. Pozos, and M. J. Buono, "An Electromyographic Approach to the Evaluation of Abdominal Exercises," *ACSM's Health & Fitness Journal* 5, no. 4 (2001): 9–14.

15. Elizabeth A. Dennis, Ana Laura Dengo, Dana L. Comber, Kyle D. Flack, Jyoti Savla, Kevin P. Davy and Brenda M. Davy, "Water Consumption Increases Weight Loss During a Hypocaloric Diet Intervention in Middle-Aged and Older Adults," *Obesity* 18: 300–307.

16. University of Texas Health Science Center at San Antonio "Waistlines in People, Glucose Levels in Mice Hint at Sweeteners' Effects: Related Studies Point to the Illusion of the Artificial," *ScienceDaily*, June 27, 2011.

17. B. C. Bullock, T. B. Clarkson, N. D. M. Lehner, H. B. Lofland Jr., R. W. St. Clair, "Atherosclerosis in Cebus albifrons monkeys: III. Clinical and Pathologic Studies," *Experimental and Molecular Pathology* 10, no. 1 (February 1969): 39–62.

Chapter 7: The 10-Minute Stretch

18. Len Kravitz, "Stretching—A Research Retrospective," *IDEA Fitness Journal*, November 2009.

19. D. Bazzett-Jones, J. B. Winchester, and J. M. McBride, "The Role of Post-Activation Potentiation and Stretching on Peak Force, Rate of Force Development, and Range of Motion in Collegiate Athletes," *Journal of Strength and Conditioning Research* 19, no. 2 (2005): 421–26.

20. M. Y. Cortez-Cooper, M. M. Anton, A. E. Devan, D. B. Neidre, J. N. Cook, and H. Tanaka, "The Effects of Strength Training on Central Arterial Compliance in Middle-Aged and Older Adults," *European Journal of Preventive Cardiology* 15, no. 2 (April 2008): 149–55.

Chapter 11: Dinner in 10 Minutes or Less

21. Primary School Lunch Provision, Centre for Food Innovation at Sheffield Hallam University, 2009, "The British Frozen Food Federation & Local Authority Caterers Association 2009 Report Frozen Foods—Use and Nutritional Acceptability."

Chapter 14: Skinny Sleep

22. National Sleep Foundation's 2008 Sleep in America poll. http://www.sleepfoundation.org/article/press-release/sleep-america-poll-summary-findings.
23. James E. Gangwisch, Dolores Malaspina, Bernadette Boden-Albala, Steven B. Heymsfield, "Inadequate Sleep as a Risk Factor for Obesity: Analyses of the NHANES," *Sleep* 28, no. 10 (Oct. 2005): 1289–96.
24. S. Taheri, L. Lin, D. Austin, T. Young, and E. Mignot, "Short Sleep Duration Is Associated with Reduced Leptin, Elevated Ghrelin, and Increased Body Mass Index," *PLoS Med* 1, no. 3 (2004).
25. Bonnefond et al, "Rare MTNR1B Variants Impairing Melatonin Receptor 1B Function Contribute to Type 2 Diabetes," *Nature Genetics* Volume: 44, no. 3 (2012): 297–301.
26. K. Spiegel, R. Leproult, M. L'Hermite-Baleriaux, G. Copinschi, P. D. Penev, and E. Van Cauter, "Leptin Levels Are Dependent on Sleep Duration: Relationships with Sympatho-Vagal Balance, Carbohydrate Regulation, Cortisol and TSH," *Journal of Clinical Endocrinology and Metabolism* 89 (2004): 5762–71.

Chapter 15: It's Not Just Physical: The Mental Side of Weight Loss

27. C. Framson, A. R. Kristal, J. M. Schenk, A. J. Littman, S. Zeliadt, and D. Benitez, "Development and Validation of the Mindful Eating Questionnaire," *Journal of the American Dietetic Association* 109, no. 8 (2009).
29. Hollis, J. American Journal of Preventive Medicine, August 2008; vol 35. Victor J. Stevens, PhD, senior investigator, Kaiser Permanente Center for Health Research, Portland, Oregon.

Index

anywhere quickies, 89
breathing during, 69, 86
increasing intensity level, 85–86
intervals, 88–100
repetitions, 85, 86
time chart, 88
Cortisol levels, 189
Cravings, dealing with, 197
Crawling plank (core exercise), 99–100
Cross tap push-ups (strength exercise), 58–59
Crunches, 85, 86, 87

D

Deep abdominal fat and walking, 26–27
Delayed onset muscle soreness (DOMS), 64–65
Depression and strength workouts, 62
Diabetes and strength workouts, 62
Diamond crunch (core exercise), 90
Diet
  effects of severe calorie restriction, 3
  recommendations, 8
Diet soda, 127
Dinner
  recipes, 148–163
  restaurant meals, 164
Double bicycle (core exercise), 93
Down & X (body circuit exercise), 77
Dumbbells, holding while walking, 36

E

Earn and burn syndrome, 8, 82
Eating
  exercising as reason for, 8, 82
  mindfully, 198–199
  sleep and, 192–193
  stress and, 199–200
  See also Restaurant meals
Encapsulation bras, 33
Equipment
  flat-belly zappers, 92
  for stretching, 107
  for 10-Minute Total Body Circuit, 70, 76, 80, 81
  for walking, 26, 33, 36–38
Exercise
  as earning food, 8, 82
  effects of dramatic increase in, 3
  intensity and weight loss, 39, 40
  intensity tracking, 40–41, 52, 55
  maintaining motivation to, 196–197
  plans for starting, 18–21
  recommendations of health organizations, 4

sleep and, 193
  "snacking" approach to, 5, 6
  stretching muscles before workouts, 103–104
  varying to overcome set points, 202
  See also specific plans
Extend & row (strength exercise), 59–60

F

Fat
  abdominal shaping and, 84
  brisk walking and, 26–27
  burning myths, 92
  high-intensity interval training and, 39
  trans fats and, 101
Fats
  controlling blood, 177–178
  olive oil, 152
Flexibility and stretching, 104, 105–106, 117
Fluids
  adequate intake of, 114
  calories in, 126, 166
  diet soda, 127
  sleep and, 192–193
Food
  allergies/intolerances, 124
  avoiding splurges, 197
  earn and burn syndrome, 8, 82
  fat-burning, 92
  importance of preparing own, 121–122
  ingredients, 126
  shopping for, 123
  substitutions to save calories, 125, 179
  trans fats, 101
  See also specific foods
Food plan
  calories based on, 124
  choices, 125
Fruits
  purchasing, 164
  as snacks, 171

G

Gherlin levels and sleep, 188
Goal setting
  form for SMART, 24
  managing expectations with, 23, 203
  SMART system, 22–23
GYMBOSS, 45

H

Heart
  benefits of stretching for, 117

About the Authors

Jessica Smith stars in several best-selling exercise DVDs, including *10 Minute Solution: Ultimate Bootcamp* and *Cross Training for Fitness* and teaches at the Miami EQUINOX Fitness Clubs and the Sports Club/LA for Canyon Ranch Hotel & Spa. She regularly contributes online to *Shape, Redbook*, and *iVillage* and writes tips and workouts for *Fitness, SELF, Shape*, and *Health* magazines. She and Liz created www.thinin10.com, an online community for thousands of women working to get their whole lives in shape.

Liz Neporent has a master's degree in fitness management from New York University. She has authored and coauthored more than a dozen best-selling health and fitness books, including *Fitness for Dummies* (Wiley, 2011) and *Weight Training for Dummies* (Wiley, 2006). She regularly contributes to numerous fitness magazines and blogs, including *Everyday Health* and *ABC News* online, *Prevention* and *More* magazines, and Dr. Oz's www.youbeauty.com.

Also Available from Sunrise River Press

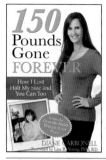

150 Pounds Gone Forever
How I Lost Half My Size and You Can Too

Diane Carbonell Mother of seven children, Diane Carbonell leads you through her journey of weight loss with real-life honesty, humor, and insight. She explains how she lost 150 pounds focusing on three simple components: fat percentage, portion control, and exercise. 150 Pounds Gone Forever shows you how to say good-bye to diets and how to change your lifestyle by identifying trigger foods, breaking unhealthy eating habits, and reorienting your thinking. The book details how to incorporate exercise into your everyday life, no matter what your weight. 6 x 9, 304 pages. Sftbd. ISBN: 978-1-934716-41-0 Item # SRP641

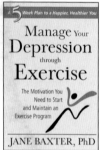

The Anti-Cancer Cookbook
How to Cut Your Risk with the Most Powerful, Cancer-Fighting Foods

Julia B. Greer, MD, MPH Dr. Julia Greer—a physician, cancer researcher, and food enthusiast—explains what cancer is and how antioxidants work to prevent pre-cancerous mutations in your body's cells, and then describes in detail which foods have been scientifically shown to help prevent which types of cancer. She shares her collection of more than 220 scrumptious recipes for soups, sauces, main courses, vegetarian dishes, sandwiches, breads, desserts, and beverages, all loaded with nutritious ingredients chock-full of powerful antioxidants that may significantly slash your risk of a broad range of cancer types, including lung, colon, breast, prostate, pancreatic, bladder, stomach, leukemia, and others. Dr. Greer even includes tips on how to cook foods to protect their valuable antioxidants and nutrients and how to make healthy anti-cancer choices when eating out. Softbound, 7.5 x 9 inches, 224 pages. Item # SRP149

2008 Midwest Book Awards Finalist!

Manage Your Depression Through Exercise
The Motivation You Need to Start and Maintain an Exercise Program

Jane Baxter, PhD Research has proven that exercise helps to lessen or even reverse symptoms of depression. Most depressed readers already know they need to exercise, but many can't muster the energy or motivation to take action. *Manage Your Depression Through Exercise* is the only book on the market that meets depressed readers where they are at emotionally, physically, and spiritually and takes them from the difficult first step of getting started toward a brighter future. Through the Move & Smile Five-Week Activity Plan, the Challenge & Correct Formula to end negative self-talk, and words of encouragement, author Jane Baxter uses facts, inspiration, compassion, and honesty to help readers get beyond feelings of inertia one step at a time. Includes reproducible charts, activities list, positive inner-dialogue comebacks, and photos illustrating various exercises. Softbound, 6 x 9 inches, 224 pages. Item # SRP624

Check Out Sunrise River Press' New, Improved Web Site!

- Find helpful tips & articles
- Get bonus material from our books
- Browse expanded e-book selections
- Look inside books before you buy
- Rate & review your Sunrise River Press collection
- Easy, user-friendly navigation
- Sign up to get e-mails with special offers
- Lightning fast, spot-on search results
- Secure online ordering
- 24/7 access

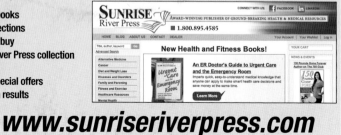

www.sunriseriverpress.com